Live Thin Live Long

By

Richard A. Uhlig, D.O.

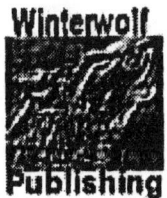

First Printing

Editing by Paula Mangino

Cover art by Kevin Grover

ISBN: 1-4196-2596-9

Additional Copies can be ordered from Amazon.com

Contents

Contents

This book is dedicated to Walter Willett, M.D. and colleagues at the Harvard School of Public Health and to the more than 50,000 health professionals who have participated in the Health Professionals Follow-up Study.

Live Thin, Live Long

CHAPTER ONE

YOU CAN TOO.

People will try almost anything to lose weight, and most of us have tried one or more of the fad diets: Low Carb Diets, Rice Diet, Protein Diet, Grapefruit Diet, Caveman Diet, Juice Diet, Sex Diet, Russian Air force Diet, Lose Six Inches off Your Belly in 8 Minutes Diet and etc. Any diet that reduces calorie intake will work in the beginning. However, after a few weeks or months, the pounds usually come back plus a few extra ones. In the meantime, you may have jeopardized your health.

Smart dieting comes down to this: the only way to lose weight, keep it off and stay healthy is to eat healthy. That's what this book is about. It's a doctor's guide to a trimmer, healthier life. It's also a disease prevention manual for longer life. If you are over 25, this book is a "must read." If you're over 50,a member of the baby boomer generation, this book could save your life.

First, beware of quick fixes that promise you'll lose 20 pounds in ten days. Watch out for diets that eliminate healthy food groups even for short periods. Avoid plans that replace meals with supplements. No safe short cuts to losing weight and keeping it off exist. Success requires lifestyle changes based on smart nutritional choices.

America is currently caught up in an "anti-carbohydrate" craze. Popular low carb diets start out by eliminating some of the very foods that keep us healthy, trim and vigorous in the long-term. Most fad diets are shortsighted, unsustainable and dieters are caught up in an endless cycle of losing, gaining and starting over. America has had enough of fad diets and recipe books that don't work and, in many instances, are unhealthy. It's time we smarten up nutritionally.

Many people embraced the "low carb" diets as "fat feasts." They gorge themselves with red meat, cheeses, eggs and other foods high in saturated fats and cholesterol, which puts them at risk for heart disease, stroke and cancer. The large amounts of protein in some of these diets may damage kidneys, especially in senior citizens and in those with high blood pressure and diabetes.

A serious flaw with many popular diets is their failure to incorporate the revolutionary findings of the Harvard Health Professionals Follow-up Study (HHPF). Even the government's food pyramid has neglected these advances in nutritional science.

I've been a participant in the HHPF since its inception 18 years ago. The findings coming out of this study are changing nutritional science rapidly. Upwards of 70% of cancers, heart attacks and strokes could be prevented if people would make healthy food choices and abstain from smoking.

The smart food choices that keep us healthy are the same ones that allow us to lose weight and keep it off. What we eat is of vital importance. Any diet or nutritional plan that ignores findings of the HHPF potentially puts the dieter at risk for a host of diseases.

This book is not a diet book in the usual sense. It's a guide to a nutritional lifestyle designed to keep you trim, energetic and mentally alert—not for six months—but for the next sixty years.

Your waistline doesn't have to bulge, your jowls don't have to sag and your get-up-and-go doesn't have to diminish just because you've turned thirty, forty, fifty, sixty, or more. You can be trimmer, healthier and, yes, even smarter, sexier and more energetic than you were ten or twenty years ago. Sounds preposterous? I've witnessed these amazing changes in my patients and in myself. There's no magic involved; it's all in what you eat.

What makes me an authority on what to eat, how to lose weight and how to stay healthy? Big city heart specialists wrote the two most popular diet books on the market and I'm just a country doctor from rural Kansas. Wouldn't cardiologists know more than a country doctor about diets? Not necessarily.

I once gave a deposition in a malpractice case that involved a heart attack patient who had a poor outcome – she died. The legal battle focused on who was at fault, the family doctor who initially cared for the patient, or the cardiologist who administered the definitive treatment. During the deposition, an attorney asked me if I agreed with his statement, "Cardiologists are better qualified to treat and advise heart patients than family doctors." I shocked the attorney when I said, "No!"

Cardiologists are busy keeping up with the explosion of technological advances in their field. After the patient receives their balloon angioplasty and stent, they're handed prescriptions for blood thinners and cholesterol pills. The cardiologist may not see them again for months or until something goes wrong.

Family doctors and I'm talking about those of us in small rural communities, are constantly in touch with our patients. We see them in the doctor's office, at the local restaurant, down at the post office and at the grocery store. We know where and how they live, we hear their complaints and we see the positive changes that occur when they take responsibility for their health. I know because I'm not only a doctor, but also a patient.

I had practiced in a small town for several years when my partner, an older doctor, unexpectedly died. I was suddenly doing the work of two doctors, delivering babies, seeing patients in the office and at the hospital and taking call seven days a week. I drank large amounts of coffee to stay awake. I smoked cigars and a pipe to ease the stress. After a few years on this frantic schedule, I decided to start exercising.

I drove to the high school football field to jog one evening. I got 50 yards down the track when pain hit me in my upper back. I kept jogging and the pain moved into my chest. "I couldn't be having a heart attack! Not me!"

The pain became excruciating and spread into my arms. I sweated as if I had run a marathon. It was late and no one around

11

to help. I managed to get to the car and drive to the hospital. The heart attack was mild. Within a week, I underwent bypass surgery. A month later, I was right back in practice, leading the same dangerous life style as before, drinking gallons of coffee and puffing on my pipe.

Eight months later, the chest pains returned. A cardiac catheterization showed my bypasses had plugged. Worse, nothing could be done surgically. There were no arteries remaining on the right side of my heart. I was surviving on small collateral arteries from the left side. I was told to go home and get along as best I could on nitroglycerin and beta-blocker medicines. I was 39 years old and I didn't think I'd see forty.

I quit smoking, which made me as edgy as a cocaine addict in withdrawal. Chewing nicotine gum loosened my dental bridges and I had to get new ones. My weight ballooned to 250 pounds and I had no control over my appetite.

For the last twenty-five years, I've studied and practiced how to stay healthy and get rid of excess pounds. I've taught others to do the same. Today my weight is in the 50th percentile, my body-mass index is less than 25 and I have no chest pains. I walk three miles four times a week, punch a punching bag daily, play basketball twice a week in the winter, swim in the summer and lift weights year around. The only medicine I take beside supplements is one-half aspirin tablet. This year I'll be old enough for Medicare.

Stress, poor food choices, excess weight and unhealthy life styles catch up with us. I know. I've been there. And I've been rescued. So can you.

*****

"Live Thin, Live Long" will teach you the smart food choices you can live with and live longer with. You'll learn strategies for handling hunger, food addiction and bad eating habits. With a little ingredient substitution, you'll turn any recipe into a healthy recipe. You'll eat your three meals a day with snacks between. You'll lose weight, keep it off and have more energy.

Starting with Chapter 2, Step Summaries at the end of each chapter allow you to quickly review the essential elements of the chapter.

Live Thin, Live Long

CHAPTER TWO

CARBOHYDRATES

After twenty-five years of chic low-fat diet advice from doctors and the media, America has gotten fatter. Almost 2/3 of the adults in the United States are overweight and 30% are obese. That is, they weigh 20% more than their ideal weight. One child in seven in America is overweight. What happened?

For the last quarter century, we replaced the fat in our diets with carbohydrates and that contributed significantly to making us overweight and unhealthy. The United States Department of Agriculture's Food Pyramid and the medical establishment are both at fault. They underestimated the role of refined carbohydrates in obesity and other health-related conditions. They compounded the problem by lumping "good" and "bad" carbohydrates together at the base of the food pyramid.

Due to the *low-carb diet* blitz, people are now cutting out all carbs and stuffing themselves with any kind of protein and fat. This happens when diets become a craze.

Restaurants with low-carb menus and grocery stores specializing in low-carb foods have popped up all over the country. Instead of cutting down on all carbs, Americans should be substituting good (healthy) carbohydrates for bad (unhealthy) carbohydrates. Eating the good carbs is essential for losing weight, keeping it off, staying healthy and living longer.

There are three basic food groups: carbohydrates, proteins and fats. Making the right food choices within each of these groups is the difference between a healthy diet that works and a fad diet that doesn't.

Carbohydrates are the most abundant food source on earth. They come from grains, vegetables and fruits. Carbohydrates are the primary ingredient in breads, pastas, cereals, sugars, honey, pastries, juices, desserts and most snack foods. They're in your salad, your casserole, your sandwich, your breakfast bagel and your soda pop. Carbohydrates make up about 50% of our daily calories and, unfortunately, most of them are refined carbohydrates — the bad ones.

Good carbs are whole grain products, fruits, and vegetables. They contain antioxidants, phytochemicals and fibers that neutralize harmful compounds, prevent accelerated aging of our tissues and organs and protect us from cancer and other diseases. They can also help keep us lose weight and stay trim. These good, health-promoting carbohydrates should never be eliminated from the diet, not even for short periods.

The *bad carbs* found in starchy foods convert rapidly to sugar when eaten, i.e. white rice, the white of potatoes and refined-grain products such as pastas, bakery goods, pretzels, breads and many cereals. "Refined" means the grain has been milled, rolled, sifted, scoured, ground, centrifuged and bleached until nearly all the important nutrients are gone. What remains is largely starch.

Starch quickly turns into sugar (glucose) in our stomachs. Glucose stimulates the production of insulin. Why is this bad? Read on.

*****

INSULIN RESISTANCE AND OBESITY

Starches are sugar molecules hooked together. When we eat starchy foods, digestion breaks the starch down into sugar molecules called glucose, which are absorbed from the stomach into the blood. The pancreas (a large gland located in the upper abdomen under the stomach) senses the increased levels of glucose in our blood and releases a hormone called insulin.

Insulin attaches to our cells and causes the glucose in our blood to enter our cells where it is burned for energy. Without insulin, we couldn't get glucose inside our cells, there would be no energy production and life would cease. When the blood glucose level drops, the pancreas stops secreting insulin and waits for the glucose level to rise again the next time we eat. Chemical messengers then tell our brains we are full. All this seems just hunky-dory. However, there are problems.

The pancreas doesn't always work smoothly, because it was not designed to handle refined carbohydrates. When we eat refined carbohydrates (white breads, white potatoes, processed cereals, white rice, donuts, pretzels, crackers and other baked goods) our blood glucose level shoots up sharply. The pancreas responds by over-secreting insulin. Excess insulin causes glucose to be changed into fat and stored in our fat cells, mainly around the belly.

Another effect of excess insulin is to make us feel hungry even though we've just eaten. If this happens often enough, we gain weight, get a fat tummy and become unhealthy.

To make things worse, weight gain causes our cells to resist insulin. When we put on excess pounds, more insulin is needed to push glucose inside our cells so it can be burned for energy. To cope with this resistance, the pancreas produces even more insulin. These higher insulin levels result in more fat being stored in our bodies, which results in more weight gain, which causes more insulin resistance. This vicious cycle leads to obesity, diabetes, high blood pressure, stroke, heart disease and even tumors.

Not all carbohydrates cause excess insulin production. Good carbs (whole grains, vegetables, fruits) break down slowly in the stomach. As a result, glucose is absorbed more slowly and this gives a smooth, even insulin response.

Loaded with fiber, antioxidants and phytochemicals, these good carbs are more filling, thus curbing the appetite and promoting loss of excess pounds. They increase our energy production and protect us from diseases. Any weight loss diet that severely limits the good carbs even for short periods gambles with the dieter's health.

Our ancestors, the cavepersons scrounged for very morsel and they didn't have refined carbohydrates to eat. They were probably thin as thistles, which was good, because they had to be quick to escape saber-tooth tigers and other menaces in the neighborhood. Obesity and insulin resistance began when human beings stopped hunting, fishing, grubbing for wild grains and berries and started farming. The human body wasn't designed to handle refined carbohydrates.

I suggest you do a "mirror test" to see if you have insulin resistance. Stand stripped in front of a full-size mirror and do both a front view and profile view of your body. If your fat is primarily located in the waist area, you have an "apple shape," meaning you either have insulin resistance or you're going to develop it. Do you have "love handles?" Then you're an apple. A "beer belly?" You're an apple. If your tummy "overhangs," or there's that "spare tire," alas, you're an apple.

Another test is to measure your abdominal girth at the narrowest point with your abdomen relaxed. For men it's at the level of the belly button. For women it's the narrowest point between the hips and breastbone. If you are a male with a girth greater than 40 inches or if you are a female with greater than 35 inches, you're an apple and you probably have insulin resistance.

If you're unsure whether you have insulin resistance, ask your doctor to check your lipids (fats in the blood). If your triglycerides are high (over a 100) and your good cholesterol called HDL is less than 35, that's a fair indication you have insulin resistance.

If your excess weight is carried in your hips and thighs, you're a "pear-shape." Pear-shapes are less prone to develop diabetes and heart disease than apples. Carbohydrates play a minor role in a "pear's" obesity.

With our epidemic of obesity in America, insulin resistance is becoming widespread. Type 2 diabetes, which was rarely seen in children before 1980, now occurs in children at an alarming rate. There is some good news. By substituting good carbs for the refined carbs, you can treat or prevent insulin resistance, take off pounds and shrink your belly. You'll lose weight and fend off a variety of diseases including diabetes.

The whole thrust of the *carbohydrate diet revolution* should be: **"Eat vegetables, fruits and whole grains and avoid refined carbs."** Sounds simple, doesn't it? Easier said than done.

Refined carbohydrates are everywhere in the American diet. Even that special Friday night dinner at that fine Italian restaurant is fraught with refined carbs. You'll need a strategy for dealing with them.

I went to my granddaughter's birthday party recently and the first words out of my daughter's mouth were, "Dad, don't start in about carbohydrates. Relax, enjoy your cake and ice cream." I did, because I've learned to have my cake and not have it too. More on strategy later. First, let's differentiate between the bad carbs that stimulate the overproduction of insulin and the good carbs that don't.

*****

REFINED CARBS VS. WHOLE GRAIN

Refined carbohydrates are white flours and processed sugars and the products made from them. These foods, which have been stripped of fiber, antioxidants and phytochemicals during processing, include many kinds of breads, cereals, bagels, donuts, cinnamon rolls, cupcakes, biscuits, French pastries, piecrust, crackers, chips, pretzels, pastas, noodles, dumplings—the list goes on. All stimulate the overproduction of insulin.

Using whole grain carbs in place of refined carbs puts you immediately on a healthy track for losing excess pounds. Eating three servings of whole grain products each day can actually lower your risk for Type II Diabetes. However, make sure what you buy is really "whole grain." Read labels and look for the words "whole grain flour."

If you don't see the word "whole" on a loaf of wheat bread, it's probably made with refined flour. Labels and advertisements are often misleading. Read the complete label as well as the ingredients. When you order "whole wheat" toast or bread at a restaurant, you're probably not going to get it. Wheat bread and whole wheat bread are not the same thing. It's a labeling trick.

Look on the grocery shelf for breakfast cereals that are 100% whole grain. Just because they have a "heart icon" on the box doesn't mean the cereal is 100% whole grain. For a product to carry the FDA's approved message that it's heart healthy, it has to contain only 51% whole grain. That's only half way. Always buy 100% whole grain products.

Most Americans overeat bread products. We eat sandwiches for both snacks and meals. We have toast in the mornings. Rolls with dinner. Crackers and croutons with salads. We should limit bread to three slices or less a day. Make sure it's whole grain— 100% with at least 3 grams of fiber per slice. Skip the crackers and croutons. If you have one serving of cereal, potato, or bakery during the day, then eliminate one slice of bread.

Only the "whole grain oatmeal," not the quick kind, gives the full dose of the healthy bran that blocks rapid sugar absorption and lowers cholesterol. It's the same with corn products, look for the words "whole grain."

When buying rice, look for the word "brown" which indicates whole grain. Wild rice can be considered whole grain. A loaf of dark rye pumpernickel on the grocery shelf is probably made with refined flour. The word "enriched" means essentially the same as refined. Again, look for the word "whole." If you like Italian food, buy whole grain pastas. Most major groceries carry them. If you're a chef or do-it-yourself gastronome, make your own zucchini or squash pasta. It's much more important to buy whole grain products than it is to buy low-carb products.

Whole grain products slow the absorption of sugar into the blood stream, preventing excess insulin responses and fat storage. Fiber, antioxidants and phytochemicals in whole grain products fend off such major problems as diabetes, heart attacks, strokes, cancer and Alzheimer's disease. Whole grain is one terrific health food bargain. Never eliminate it from your diet.

GLYCEMIC INDEX

The glycemic index (GI) is a measure of how rapidly an ingested food causes blood sugar to rise. Generally, the faster it rises, the more erratic and excessive will be the insulin response. Foods are ranked on the glycemic scale, ranging from 0 to 100. Many scales arbitrarily assign a score of 100 to pure sugar (glucose). Foods high on the G.I. scale (greater than 60) stimulate excess insulin production and overuse can lead to insulin resistance. Foods low on the scale have a milder effect on insulin production.

Fruit juices have a high G.I. and are not much better than soda pop for controlling insulin levels and for losing weight. A baked potato has a whopping G.I. of 85. Blueberries, on the other hand, are packed with anti-oxidants and have a GI of less than 50. Any food with a G.I. over 75 should raise a red flag, e.g. potatoes, candied fruits, parsnips, dried bananas, dates, pretzels, corn flakes, French fries, jelly beans, waffles, corn chips, hamburger and hot dog buns.

Apples, oranges and berries have much lower G.I.s than bananas, kiwi and grapes. The GI isn't a perfect indication of whether a carb is good or bad. Grapes have a GI higher than some milk puddings. Red or darkly colored grapes are packed with antioxidants and should never be totally excluded from your diet. Puddings can be excluded without any health risk. At best, the Glycemic Index is a reference guide.

GLYCEMIC INDEX OF COMMON FOODS

dates	100
white bread	95
instant rice	87
baked potato	85

corn flakes	85
pretzels	82
rice cakes	82
carrots	75
puffed wheat	74
saltines	74
watermelon	72
beets	70
taco shells	68
angel food cake	67
sweet potato	60
popcorn	55
grapes	50
apple	40
tomato	38
yogurt	35
peach	30
green beans	30
kidney beans	27
grapefruit	25
peanuts	10

The above is a sampling of the Glycemic Index from a composite of indices. More detailed listings are available on the World Wide Web.

How much carbohydrate should a person consume in a day? This varies with your size, metabolism and energy needs. Apple-shapes and obese individuals should sharply limit their carbs to roughly 120 grams a day. Most Americans consume twice that much. A cup of skim milk has 12 grams, a slice of bread is 12 grams, a large bagel about 50 grams, a serving of pasta 40 grams and green beans 4 grams. It's more important to substitute whole grain for refined carbs than it is to count grams.

Some common sense rules for limiting carbs are: if you have cereal for breakfast, leave off the toast. Don't eat cereal and pasta on the same day. If lunch includes a sandwich, omit any bakery products that day. Sugar, juice, soda pop, potatoes (with the exception of sweet potatoes), white rice, chips, fries and sugary treats may be considered refined carbs and should be sharply limited. When it comes to carbs, go "whole grain."

FRUITS AND VEGETABLES

Fruits and vegetables along with whole grain products make up the good carbs. An adult should eat at least seven to nine servings of fruits and vegetables a day. A serving size for raw vegetables is about one cup; for cooked vegetables, ½ cup; for fruit, ½ cup; for dried fruit, 1/4 cup.

Fruit and vegetables supply the majority of our vitamins, antioxidants and phytochemicals. As a rule, the more deeply colored the fruit or vegetable, the healthier. With few exceptions, fruit and vegetables have G.I.s below 70 and their effect on insulin levels is minor compared to refined carbs. The exceptions are watermelon and carrots, which, despite the high GI's, are chuck full of health-promoting nutrients.

Fruit juices have a whopping 40 grams of carbs per serving, most of it in the form of sugar. Juice drinks are often sweetened with corn syrup, another form of sugar that promotes excess pounds. When you drink juice instead of eating the fruit, you don't get the health-promoting fiber and only a portion of the antioxidants and phytochemicals. It's better to skip the juice and go for the "pulpy" real stuff. Eating whole vegetables and fruit prevents excessive insulin levels, fat deposition and weight gain.

Green vegetables supply folic acid, which is important in preventing colon cancer and heart disease. Spinach contains health-promoting omega-3 fatty acids and antioxidants that protect the eyes.

Tomatoes are rich in lycopene, a gladiator against prostate, esophageal and breast cancers. Lycopene also protects against macular degeneration, a common cause of blindness. Cooked tomatoes have more available lycopene than raw tomatoes. Tomato paste and sauces are rich sources of lycopene. Watermelon, despite its high G.I., is an excellent source of lycopene.

Studies indicate broccoli and cabbage are beneficial in preventing bladder cancer and other malignancies of the urinary tract. I recommend eating broccoli every day. Broccoli sprouts have more anti-cancer properties than mature broccoli. Quick freezing of vegetables and fruits seals in the phytochemicals and antioxidants and reduces the need for preservatives.

A study done by the Harvard School of Public Health, funded by the NHI and published in the Journal of the American Medical Association showed eating a mere six servings of fruit and vegetables a day reduced the risk for brain stroke by 30%. Vegetarians have less heart disease and cancer than non-vegetarians and some studies show they live longer — a powerful endorsement for eating your fruit and vegetables.

STEP 1: REPLACE REFINED CARBOHYDRATES WITH WHOLE GRAIN PRODUCTS. AVOID SUGARY SNACKS AND SUGARY SOFT DRINKS.
STEP 2: IF YOU HAVE CEREAL FOR BREAKFAST, LEAVE OFF THE TOAST.
STEP 3: DON'T EAT CEREAL AND PASTA ON THE SAME DAY.
STEP 4: DON'T EAT A SANDWICH AND PASTRY ON THE SAME DAY.
STEP 5: EAT 7 TO 9 OR MORE SERVINGS OF FRUIT AND VEGETABLES A DAY

Richard A. Uhlig, D.O.

CHAPTER THREE

STRATEGIES

To lose those excess pounds and keep them off, you need to get through those "eating situations" that can derail a healthy lifestyle.

Holiday dinners, family reunions, church socials, picnics, chamber of commerce dinners, Aunt Myrtle's Sunday specials and other gala events occur regularly in our lives. When counted up, these special times can sink any diet for the entire year. The secret is to enjoy them while keeping your nutritional lifestyle on track. At these wonderful life-affirming events, don't make food the main attraction.

The most dangerous diet period of the year, when most pounds accumulate, starts at Halloween and ends on New Year's Day. Some people gain 20 pounds during this time and then spend the rest of the year trying to lose it.

Here is what you can do about it: if you're on an exercise program, increase the time, the miles, the sessions during this period. Don't skip any sessions. If you're not on an exercise program, start one. Give up a special holiday food during this period: turkey, cake, fudge—something you know you usually over-indulge in.

Write down everything you eat during the holidays: meals, snacks, treats—everything. Merely writing it down will keep most people on track. Lastly, each night look at the foods and amounts you've taken in. You'll do better the next day.

My son taught me an eating trick when he was in seventh

grade. Junior High students dined under the watchful eye of a haranguing lunchroom monitor who blew up whenever they didn't eat their hotdog and bun, mashed potatoes covered in white gravy, cake and whole milk.

My son hated hotdogs. To avoid being scolded, he chopped up his hotdog and mixed it with the other foods on his plate to give it a mutilated 'having-been-partaken-of' appearance. Squirting ketchup, sometimes the only vegetable on the table, over the whole mess, he kept the monitor guessing.

Use this trick at those community social functions like church dinners and the county's Annual Historical Society Dinner, where everybody is served the same suicidal menu. In my town, it's fired meat smothered in brown gravy, mashed or baked potato, sweetened can fruit in jiggling green Jell-O and oven-fresh rolls that send insulin levels through the ceiling. Usually there's a salad and for dessert a cake with pink sugar icing.

While you visit with your neighbors at the table, sip water and start tearing your roll to pieces. While the others eat, quietly rip apart your food with your fork and knife. Once it's well shredded, meld it together with the spoon and move it around. Hide the fried meat under the mashed potatoes and use the roll's remains to sop up the gravy. At first, you'll feel like a food sadist, but you'll get used to it. No one will notice.

If you get bored sitting there while everyone is eating, mix the condiments together and turn your plate into something Jackson Pollock-sque. You can get through an entire dangerous meal by eating the salad (watch out for the dressing—it could be loaded). Eat only the skin of the baked potato, that's where the vitamins and minerals are stashed. The rest of the potato consists of starch, which immediately turns to sugar in the stomach.

It doesn't take will power? The trick is to eat before you go to the dinner and have a healthy snack when you get home.

*****

Years ago, I saw a movie about a Swedish ship captain and his crew who were smuggling a scientist out of Nazi Germany. They knew their small ship would be stopped and searched on the North Sea. The captain planned to get the Nazi patrol guards drunk while he and his crew stayed sober. He drank a cup of mineral oil made palatable with a little cheese, then ordered his crew to do likewise.

When the Nazis came on board, the captain offered them whiskey. Then the captain and his crew drank and joked with the Nazis late into the night. The Nazis became so drunk they forgot to search the ship. The captain and his crew remained sober, because the mineral oil had slowed the absorption of whiskey from their stomachs.

The story has a strong element of truth. Fats and oils slow the absorption of not only alcohol but sugar from the intestinal tract into the blood stream, preventing excessive insulin responses. Taking some fat with your pasta or bread is a good idea. Make sure it's a healthy fat (see the next chapter), and that the bread is whole grain.

Fiber, protein foods and acids found in some salad dressings also slow the absorption of glucose. If you use fiber for this purpose, use a soluble fiber like bran or pectin found in whole grain oats and apples.

A teaspoon of antioxidant-rich grape seed oil, a fish oil capsule, or a flaxseed oil capsule before a carb-rich meal is a good method of smoothing out insulin spikes. Grape seed oil contains linoleic acid, which lowers bad cholesterol and raises good cholesterol.

Fish oil and flaxseed oil are rich in health-promoting omega-3 fatty acid. I recommend taking a fish oil capsule before meals to lessen the insulin surges. Fish oil is one of the healthiest food supplements around. We'll talk more about that in the next chapter.

When Italian restaurants coat their spaghetti with olive oil, they're doing you a favor. Your stomach turns spaghetti into glucose and the olive oil slows the absorption of the glucose, preventing an excessive insulin response. Remember, high insulin levels cause the deposition of fat around the belly and sets you up for diabetes and other morbid conditions.

I know it seems counter-intuitive that fats and oils protect one from gaining weight, but it's true. The secret is using a healthy "good" fat to do the job. Also don't overuse.

Before going to my granddaughter's birthday party, I swallowed a fish oil capsule, drank a large glass of water and ate a slice of soy cheese. At the party, I was served the proverbial ice cream and cake on a disposable plastic plate. Incidentally, if you must eat one or the other, pick the ice cream over the cake. The sugar in ice cream is absorbed much slower than the sugar in the cake.

Standing on the patio midst the brightly colored helium balloons, I mutilated the cake and whirled the ice cream with my plastic spoon. Then, after the ice cream melted, I dumped the whole mess into a trash container. I stayed socially involved the whole time. My daughter was delighted I hadn't opened my mouth about refined carbs to spoil the fun.

No one wants to go through life missing the desserts. You can make a healthy, nutritious cake using whole gain flour, healthy oils and egg whites. Or, you can replace half the oil in the recipe with applesauce. In place of icing, top your cake with fruit. Buy low fat cake mixes.

Watch out for the piecrusts, most are fattening and unhealthy. I found lard and trans fats in all the commercially available piecrusts in a survey of local grocery stores in my area. You can make a healthy piecrust using whole grain flour and ground almonds. Substitute frozen fat-free yogurt, soy ice cream, or sherbet for regular ice cream.

Going to the movies can be dangerous to your health? Many theater chains still pop the popcorn in saturated oil. Add butter and you got a saturated fat bomb in a box. Add soda pop, some Gummi Bears or M&M's and the only thing that can possibly save you is a stomach pump. If the movies aren't considerate enough to pop their corn in healthy oil, then smuggle in a sack of home-popped corn. Take along some bottled water. You'll save money and anywhere from 1000 to 3000 calories and you'll be trimmer and healthier for the effort. You won't go to jail if you're caught.

*****

PITCHFORK OR SCOOP

Like an avid birdwatcher, I observe people eating. I do it at social dinners, restaurants, the hospital cafeteria and at picnics. I try not to be conspicuous and make a point not to stare. Having spent much of my youth on a farm pitching hay and scooping grain, I found the pitchfork and scoop to be useful analogies for "types of eaters."

The *SCOOP EATERS*, usually overweight, scoop the food in. They lean over the table, mouth near plate, sometimes an arm curled around the plate and scoop until their cheeks bulge. They talk very little and rarely put down their eating utensils. Sometimes their eyes glaze and they seemed to be daydreaming as they eat.

The *PITCHFORK EATERS* usually sit erect, stab at their food and put no more than a one-fork morsel into their mouths at a time. They put down the eating utensil frequently, chew slowly and talk more. Pitchfork eaters are usually thinner and healthier-looking. It'd behoove us all to become pitchforkers. We have many opportunities to practice, at least three times a day.

*****

THE TWENTY-MINUTE LAG

Since our ancient ancestors, the cave people, aren't around to defend themselves, we can blame them for our bad eating habits.

When feasting on a felled mammoth or some other hard-won prize, they probably gorged themselves even after their stomachs were full. It was a survival strategy. They knew their next meal could be days or weeks away.

After a full, delicious meal, while the digestive juices are still flowing and the taste buds are still tingling, we often get the urge to eat more. We know better. We're not hungry, but the urge is compelling.

Wait a minute—well, twenty minutes.

Reach down inside and pull out a little will power. Look at your watch and promise yourself that you'll not take another bite of food for twenty minutes. Take a walk, read, or watch TV— get involved in something for twenty minutes. Usually, the taste buds stop tingling and the food urge passes. If the urge persists, drink a full glass of water, then give yourself a small treat like a little piece of dark chocolate, some peanuts, or a few grapes.

*****

ORGANIC FOODS

The Department of Agriculture ensures organic foods are grown, harvested and processed according to strict standards. You can have confidence in the "Organic" label.

By eating organic, you decrease your exposure to pesticides and avoid foods that have been irradiated, treated with manure, sewage by-products and synthetic fertilizers. Recently, an outbreak of hepatitis A on the East Coast was attributed to green onions, which may have been grown with a fertilizer containing human waste.

Every chance you get, go organic. Especially for those foods that often contain high levels of pesticide residues: apples, peaches, peppers, green beans and green onions. Organic is good for you and the environment. The downside is that it may cost more and organic may not be readily available in your area.

STEP 6: TAKE A FISH OIL CAPSULE BEFORE MEALS.
STEP 7: EAT BEFORE GOING TO SOCIAL DINNERS, AND EAT A HEALTHY SNACK WHEN YOU GET HOME.
STEP 8: BE A PITCHFORK EATER.
STEP 9: GIVE YOURSELF TWENTY MINUTES FOR A FOOD URGE TO PASS.

Richard A. Uhlig, D.O.

CHAPTER FOUR

THE THICK AND THIN OF FATS

For the last twenty years, fats have taken a beating. Clogged arteries have fat in them. Obese people have too much stored fat. Americans went overboard and eliminated both the bad and good fats from their diets. Consequently, America got fatter. The pendulum has swung back and fats are now the vogue.

Beware!

With the low-carb diet books, came "fat" advocates extolling virtues of fatty foods and doling out heavy recipes *carte blanche*. The pendulum has swung too far. Today, both bad carbs and bad fats are making us overweight and unhealthy. Again, getting trim and staying healthy comes down to smart food choices. We must discern the "good" fats from the "bad fats."

Many confusing chemical terms are used to describe fats. There are three main types: saturated fats, trans fats and unsaturated fats. Saturated fats and trans fats are the bad guys.

Saturated fats are found in many foods and are solid at room temperature (lard, shortenings and animal fats). Food manufacturers produce trans fats by adding hydrogen to liquid oils to thicken them, hence the names "hydrogenated" and "partially hydrogenated." Saturated fats and trans fats are associated with heart attacks, strokes and other health risks. Eating these fats raises the bad (LDL) cholesterol levels in the blood and lowers good (HDL) cholesterol levels, a situation that leads to clogged arteries.

Major dietary sources of saturated fats are red meat (pork, beef, lamb) and dairy products (milk, cheese, butter). Two percent milk is not low fat. Use skim milk to cut down on the artery-clogging saturated fat. Skim milk is the best dairy buy on the market and contains more calcium than whole milk.

To further cut down on saturated fat, use only lean cuts of meat, no more than 3 to 6 ounces in any one day and trim off all visible fat. Or use chicken, fish, turkey, or soy products for main dishes. Vegetable sources of saturated fat are palm oil, coconut and coca butter.

Unsaturated fats are thin fats, liquid at room temperature (olive oil, most vegetable oils, and fish oil). Unsaturated fats help keep us trim, healthy, smart and they even fight depression. There are two types: monounsaturated and polyunsaturated. These unsaturated fats are the good guys. In the confusing world of fat nomenclature, the "UN" (just think of the United Nations) fats are the good guys. Remember, the UNsaturated fats are the healthy ones.

Unfortunately, food manufacturers add bad trans fats to all kinds of foods: crackers, cookies, chips, peanut butter, snack items, salad dressings, margarines, bakery goods, cereals, French fries and fast food cuisine.

Ideally, one should cut out trans fats completely, but they are so ubiquitous, you can only strive to keep consumption as low as possible. Trans fats can be identified on food labels by the phrase, "made with hydrogenated oil" or "made with partially hydrogenated oil."

One way to avoid bad fats is to avoid deep fried foods. French fries are a no-no. When eating a salad leave off the crackers and croutons are use the low fat croutons. Watch out for frozen pizza, potpies, snack foods of all kinds and breaded fish sticks—read those labels. Choose breakfast cereals with the least amount of saturated fat and avoid those made with trans fats. Look through your refrigerator and kitchen pantry; you'll be amazed at all the products containing trans fats (hydrogenated or partially hydrogenated oils).

*****

Peanut butter is an excellent snack food; a tablespoon between meals can alleviate hunger. Peanut butter contains the antioxidant resveratrol, which extends the natural life of yeast cells and may do the same for human cells. However, many peanut butter products contain "hydrogenated" or "partially hydrogenated oils" to thicken it. To avoid these bad fats use "natural" peanut butter. The pure peanut oil in natural peanut butter is so thin it floats at the top of the jar, but refrigeration firms it up.

The Food and Drug Administration has required food manufacturers to list amounts of trans fats in their products by 2006. Until then, it's buyer beware and read the labels.

New cholesterol-lowering spreads like Take Control and Benecol offer a considerable advantage over the trans-fat margarines. Made from plant stanols and sterols, these spreads have a healthy ratio of unsaturated to saturated fat and they bind cholesterol in the digestive tract, preventing it from getting into the bloodstream.

When it comes to fats, you are in the thick and thin of a food war. READ YOUR FOOD LABELS! Avoid trans fats (hydrogenated or partially hydrogenated) whenever possible. Keep saturated fats to a minimum. Stick with the health-promoting "UN" fats found in nuts, fruits, vegetables, fish and other seafoods. Use vegetable oils when preparing foods.

*****

CHOLESTEROL

Cholesterol is not a fat, but has physical properties that resemble fats. Our cells use cholesterol to make hormones, vitamin D and other essential substances. A high cholesterol level is a risk factor for clogged arteries and thus for heart attacks and strokes. Our livers manufacture cholesterol, especially when we consume saturated fats and trans fats. We also get cholesterol directly from foods we eat.

Cholesterol exists in two forms in our bodies, good (high density) and bad (low density). The high-density cholesterol (HDL) actually protects us from heart attacks.

Have your cholesterol levels checked by your doctor. Generally, your total cholesterol should be less than 200 milligrams. The high density (HDL) cholesterol should be 35 or higher, the higher the better. Keep your bad cholesterol (LDL) below 130, the lower the better. If you already have heart disease or plugged arteries, keep it 60 or below. Check with your doctor. Remember trans fats and saturated fats raise your cholesterol.

The soluble fiber in nuts, apples, beans, whole grain oats, peas and other vegetables and fruits bind cholesterol in the stomach and prevent it from being absorbed into the blood. Soluble fiber also prevents bile salts in the intestines from being reabsorbed and converted into cholesterol.

Tips for controlling Cholesterol: When preparing chicken, remove the skin. Use only lean cuts of meat and strip away all the fat. Increase fish in your diet, especially salmon. Use soy products. Roast or bake instead of frying. Drink skim milk or soymilk in place of whole milk. Use low-fat cheese or soy cheese. As mentioned earlier, use Benecol or Take Control instead of margarine spreads containing trans fats.

*****

TRIGLYCERIDES

Triglyceride is another fat that clogs arteries. If you are an apple-shape with insulin resistance, or a diabetic, or have a family history of diabetes, you probably have elevated triglycerides. Eating refined carbs increases triglycerides in the blood. Avoiding refined carbs, trans fats and saturated fats will help reduce your triglyceride level. Your doctor may prescribe a medication if your triglycerides are too high. Aim to keep your triglyceride level below 100.

*****

OMEGA FATTY ACIDS

Two types of fatty acids called omega-3 and omega-6 play vital roles in the health and normal functioning of our cells. Maintaining the right balance between these fatty acids is crucial. When correctly balanced, these fatty acids may reduce your risk for heart disease, high blood pressure and breast cancer.

Our caveperson ancestors ate wild animals, fish and nuts, which are rich in omega-3 fatty acid and omega-6. Today the situation is different. We get plenty of omega-6 from eating grain-fed livestock, wheat, corn, rice cereals and foods containing canola oil, safflower oil and sunflower oil. We don't get enough omega-3 and this throws us out of balance.

Fish oil can increase your omega-3. Flaxseed oil is also a good source of omega-3, but it also contains some omega-6 and omega-9. Salmon, mackerel, tuna, green leafy vegetables and walnuts are rich in omega-3 fatty acids.

I've prescribed fish oil to heart patients since the 1970's. Back then, we had no idea it also helped cool the inflammation of arthritis and reduced the risk for some cancers. Recent research suggests that taking fish oil may help depression and migraines. Many people are concerned about mercury levels in fish and rightly so. However, mercury is water soluble and probably not found in high levels in fish oil. However, mercury contamination is a legitimate concern and more research needs to be done.

Fish oil or flaxseed oil is an essential daily supplement to anyone eating a modern diet.

*****

COCONUT OIL

Some nutritionists tout coconut oil as a health food and an aid to weight-loss. Coconuts contain saturated fats and even though these fatty acids are rapidly absorbed and metabolized, they're still saturated fats. In the past heart-patients have been told to avoid coconut. Coconut does contain lauric acid, which some researchers think may help heart disease. The jury is still out. At present, I don't recommend using coconut oil.

STEP 10: USE ONLY LEAN CUTS OF RED MEAT, NO MORE THAN 3 to 6 OUNCES IN ANY ONE DAY. TRIM AWAY ALL FAT. AVOID PROCESSED MEATS. USE CHICKEN, FISH, OR TURKEY AS MAIN DISHES.

STEP 11: USE SOY MILK OR SKIM MILK IN PLACE OF WHOLE MILK OR 2% MILK.

STEP 12: USE LOW-FAT OR FAT-FREE CHEESE OR SOY-CHEESE.

STEP 13: ROAST OR BAKE INSTEAD OF FRYING. NEVER DEEP-FRY.

STEP 14: READ THOSE LABELS. AVOID TRANS FATS. REDUCE SATURATED FATS TO A MINIMUM.

CHAPTER FIVE

PROTEINS

Let's take a minute to review. Eating refined carbohydrates raises insulin levels, which results in fat deposition and weight gain, which can lead to insulin resistance, obesity and health problems. Most crackers, pretzels, pastas, breads and baked goods are made with refined carbohydrates. Potatoes, white rice and chips are also high on the G.I. scale.

We learned that ingesting a little unsaturated oil, protein, or fiber before meals can blunt insulin spikes.

We should use whole grain products in place of refined carbs and eat 7 to 9 servings of fruits and vegetables every day. We know that the good "**UN**" fats keep us healthy, while the bad saturated and trans fats (hydrogenated and partially hydrogenated) are associated with heart attacks, strokes and other problems. Used daily as a supplement, fish oil or flax seed oil are good sources of health-promoting omega-3 fatty acids.

We've looked at strategies for turning down foods we shouldn't be eating without appearing unsociable. We've stepped around some food traps and are on our way to sliming down and becoming healthier.

After just a week of avoiding refined carbs and bad fats, you'll begin to lose your craving for starchy foods and carb snacks. You'll feel more energetic and notice your belly is shrinking. Before long, you'll start getting into those clothes at the back of the closet. You may notice a mild constipation. Usually this will remedied itself.

Any persistent change in bowel habits requires a checkup by your doctor.

Now for the proteins.

*****

Proteins are amino acids (compounds containing carbon and nitrogen) strung together into long chains. Proteins are the workhorses of our bodies: the muscles that give us movement, the enzymes that drive metabolism, the antibodies that fight invading germs, the hormones that regulate function and the hemoglobin that transports oxygen in the blood. Proteins also form the scaffolding of our bodies, which give us shape and strength.

The human body can't make all the amino acids it needs, so we must get some of them directly from the foods we eat. Animal protein sources include beef, lamb, pork, poultry, fish, shellfish, eggs and milk products. Human beings can use virtually any animal protein. In some countries, horsemeat is a source of protein. In others, dogs. In parts of Asia, boiled cats are a protein delicacy. Goat meat is popular in the Middle East.

Plant protein sources are: nuts, grains, legumes (beans, peas, lentils, and peanuts), fruits and vegetables. Proteins cannot be stored in our bodies. When they break down, we need to replenish them.

Protein deficiency is almost unheard of in the United States, and there is little need for high-protein supplements. When excess protein is broken down, the nitrogen from protein is excreted by the kidneys. Kidney function decreases with age, about 1% per year after age 30. Excess protein intake can tax the kidneys of those us over 50.

From childhood, most of us were given meat and dairy as our primary protein source and we have under-used fish, poultry and vegetable protein sources. A healthy protein source contains healthy fats. Vegetables provide quality protein as well as healthy unsaturated fats, fiber, phytochemicals, vitamins and antioxidants.

Nuts, soy, fish, whole grains and legumes are excellent sources of healthy protein.

*****

SALMON

Salmon is one of the best protein food choices available. The protein, exceptionally lean and high quality, provides all the essential amino acids (those our bodies cannot make). Salmon is replete with B vitamins, vitamin A, vitamin D, zinc, magnesium, phosphorus and coenzyme Q-10 antioxidant. The fat in salmon is polyunsaturated and includes health-promoting omega-3 fatty acids. As a bonus, salmon is rich in DMAE, dimethylaminoethanol, the brain food. DMAE is purported to help memory and to lessen skin wrinkles.

Levels of contaminants such as mercury are usually lower in wild salmon compared to some other coldwater fish. Mercury poisoning is serious, particularly in pregnant women (causes brain damage in the fetus as well as adults). PCBs, pesticides, dioxin and other chemicals also pose a risk for fish eaters.

If you eat lot of fish and are in doubt about your mercury status, have your doctor order a blood mercury level. I eat only wild salmon and not farm-raised salmon. Unfortunately, a survey of restaurants in my area showed they all served only farm-raised salmon. So, I eat home-cooked, wild Alaskan salmon.

Sardines are a good food choice, but I recommend eating them only once a week or less because of the risk of toxins. All other fish, I eat only rarely and that includes shrimp and tuna. I've stopped eating snapper and white albacore tuna because of mercury. Unfortunately, some of our healthiest food choices have become tainted by pollution.

A study done at Rush Presbyterian-St. Luke's Medical Center in Chicago showed a 60% reduction in the risk of Alzheimer's disease in those that ate fish once a week compared to those who never ate fish. Another study showed that eating fish once per month or more reduced the risk of stroke in men.

I recommend eating wild salmon twice a week or more. If you don't like the fishy taste or smell, cut the salmon fillets into small pieces and simmer them in bouillon or chicken broth with a mixture of vegetables. When broiling salmon, cover fillets with lemon juice before broiling and add oregano, dill, marjoram, tarragon, or a combination of these to the finished product. Use a low calorie tartar sauce, look for one that isn't spiked with high-fructose corn syrup.

Try a salmon burger. Cut the salmon into chunks and throw it into a food processor along with some basil sauce and pepper. Work the processed salmon into burger patties and grill them or brown them in the skillet using a little olive oil spray. Top them with salsa or a tomato relish. Use whole grain bread or a whole grain tortilla wrap instead of buns. You'll get a healthy burger without the fish taste.

Mix your processed salmon with couscous and your favorite spices and top it with tomato paste, bake it in a bread pan—you'll end up with a healthy, great tasting meatloaf.

*****

SOY

Soy is a complete protein (contains all the essential amino acids). Soy promotes health by lowering "bad" LDL cholesterol. Low fat soy foods can reduce the risk of heart disease.

For years, we doctors prescribed estrogen pills to women with hot flashes and softening of the bones. Because estrogen is associated with an increase risk of cancer of the uterus, progesterone, another hormone was added to it. Touted to be a preventive for heart disease and Alzheimer's, these hormone products were prescribed to increasing numbers of post-menopausal women. Recent studies show that hormones actually had the opposite effects on the heart and brain and put women at risk for the very diseases they were trying to prevent.

Whether or not to take hormones to control menopausal symptoms is complicated question and should be discussed with your doctor. I personally don't recommend them.

Soy contains phytoestrogens (plant estrogens), which may cool down hot flashes and in theory block estrogen's effect on the breast, which some think should reduce the risk of breast cancer. Studies are underway to test soy's effect on menopause symptoms and breast cancer.

I recommend soy as a regular source of protein. Soy comes in many forms. Tofu is soy curd and is great in an omelet and with many other foods. I've even made soy fudge using tofu and semi-sweet dark chocolate. Soymilk can be used just like cow's milk. Tempeh has the texture of meat. Miso is a soy paste. Soy flour and powder can be used for baking.

Soy burgers, soy hotdogs and other soy products resembling meat dishes are available in the frozen food section of the grocery. Soy cheeses taste good and come in the traditional cheese flavors. Asians, whose diets are high in soy, have lower rates of heart disease, obesity, breast cancer and prostate cancer than Americans.

*****

EGGS

Eggs are another source of complete protein. The white of the egg contains the protein; the yellow (yolk) contains fat. The fat is mostly polyunsaturated with about 200 milligrams of cholesterol.

Make sure your eggs are cooked "done." Wash your hands when handling uncooked eggs and broken eggshells. Salmonella poisoning kills a number of people every year and you never know which egg might be contaminated. Thorough cooking destroys Salmonella.

Eating egg whites is an excellent way to get your protein without the fat. To cut down on calories, use egg whites instead of whole eggs in pastries, mixes, omelets, etc. Egg yolks should be limited to two a week, or leave them off entirely. If you like a yellow color to your scrambled eggs, try the yolk-free commercial products such as "Egg Beaters."

*****

NUTS

Nuts are an excellent source of protein. Peanuts, which are actually legumes, are about a quarter protein, which is more protein per ounce than eggs and fish. We've already mentioned that peanuts are rich in resveratrol. Walnuts, a source of omega-3 fatty acids, also contain ellagic acid, thought to be a cancer inhibitor. Brazil nuts provide selenium, another anti-cancer chemical. Almonds are an excellent source of vitamin E, the protein is high quality and the fat unsaturated. Nuts are being researched for a host of health benefits including the prevention of abnormal heart rhythms.

A handful of nuts make an excellent snack. When eating nuts most of us have a tendency to overdo. Use unsalted nuts and make sure no hydrogenated or partially hydrogenated oils have been added to the product. Nuts go well in salads and add texture and flavor to many foods. Before leaving the basic food groups, we need to mention a few other important nutrients.

*****

WATER

Water is a health food and an essential nutrient. We can't live more than 2 to 3 days without it. Most of us don't take in enough.

Drink at least 6 to 9 glasses of water a day depending on your size and activity level. Drink an extra glass for every 20 pounds over ideal weight. Drink more when you exercise. A good formula is one or two glasses an hour before exercise, a ½ glass every 15 minutes during exercise and another one or two glasses afterwards. If you exercise vigorously, you'll need more water.

Drink a glass of water every morning to jumpstart the day. Don't substitute soft drinks, coffee and tea for water. The diuretic effects of these drinks can cause the body to lose water. You should have that glass of water in addition to your morning coffee.

Our bodies are 2/3 water and our brains are 80% water. That's why people become giddy and confused when dehydrated. To be at your best for an athletic contest, business meeting, interview, or an exam, stay hydrated.

Water is also an anti-cancer nutrient. Water flushes carcinogens from our bodies. Drinking more water and urinating frequently reduces contact time between carcinogens in the urine and the bladder wall, reducing the risk of bladder cancer. Don't hold back. Empty your bladder when you feel the urge.

Tap water in the United States has been considered safe. However, our government considered down-regulating arsenic levels in drinking water. Arsenic is a cancer-causing contaminant formed as a by-product of copper smelting and the combustion of low-grade coal. It's also a poison. What were they thinking?

MTBE, a gasoline additive, has contaminated drinking water in many communities and the government is taking little or no action to prevent it. Write your congressional representative about the need for stricter regulation of these dangerous substances.

Under the Safe Drinking Water Act, water companies are required to list contaminant levels once a year for customers. They often hide the bad news about contaminants deep within the report, or they fail to send out the report to consumers. If you didn't receive a report, call the company or the Environmental Protection Agency and demand one.

Check your water report for the following contaminants: **Lead** — causes neurological damage in children under six. **Arsenic,**

Asbestos, Atrazine, Benzene, and Perchlorate — can cause cancer. **Nitrates** from fertilizers — -affects the blood of small children and can cause miscarriages and birth defects. **Mercury** — causes brain damage, especially in developing infants, but also in adults.

Main source of mercury contamination is coal burning power plants. Unfortunately, the oceans are even contaminated with mercury. The FDA and EPA have issued warnings to women about eating certain kinds of fish contaminated with mercury.

Women in their childbearing years should avoid shark, king mackerel, and tilefish. Albacore tuna has been reported as having more mercury than canned light tuna. Check with your state government about the safety of fresh water fish in your area.

Keeping our water safe, keeps us healthy. If you believe your water supply is unsafe, drink distilled bottled water.

*****

FIBER

Fiber is the indigestible part of plants. There are two varieties: soluble and insoluble. Soluble fiber binds cholesterol and prevents it from being absorbed from the stomach. It also slows the absorption of sugar, blunting insulin spikes. Whole grain carbs, apples and vegetables are good sources of soluble fiber.

Insoluble fiber relieves constipation, reduces your risk for developing diverticulosis (pockets in the colon) and hemorrhoids. Insoluble fiber may play a role in preventing colon cancer by binding up and rapidly eliminating carcinogens (cancer causing chemicals).

Eating high fiber foods gives us a full feeling, which helps curb the appetite. Food labels list only total fiber. Most whole grain, vegetable, and fruit sources are a mixture of both types. We need about 25 to 40 grams of fiber a day.

*****

ARTIFICIAL SWEETENERS

I haven't seen any proof that artificial sweeteners help in losing weight and many people feel the safety issues concerning these products have not been fully resolved. These chemicals can cause gas and diarrhea in some people. Young children, pregnant women and nursing mothers should not use saccharine. People with Phenylketonuria, PKU, should not use aspartame (NutraSweet).

Non-caloric sweeteners have a place in controlling diabetes in some patients. However, just because you've been diagnosed with diabetes doesn't mean you automatically have to use artificial sweeteners. It's an old medical yarn that diabetics should never eat table sugar. Actually, it's not the sugar, but the how much of it you use that's important. Table sugar is just another refined carb and has a lower G.I. than the potato. If you eat something sugary, then cut out a starchy food.

I prefer to use small amounts of dark honey in lieu of artificial sweeteners. The polyphenols in dark honey (such as buckwheat honey) are potent antioxidants that protect the human body from many degenerative processes.

In the last two decades, food manufacturers have been putting *high fructose corn syrup* in all sorts of products to sweeten them up. This additive is in ketchup, soda pop, tartar sauce, juices, bakery goods, candy, (even wholesome whole wheat bread); it's in nearly everything, but it's not in your best interest.

Fructose is a natural sugar. Through a mechanism probably unrelated to insulin resistance, fructose can make us fat. Again, it's not that fructose itself is bad (it occurs naturally in honey and fruits), it's that we're getting so much of it in so many different kinds of foods.

You can cut down on fructose by not drinking soda pop, juices and juice drinks that have corn syrup added. Use fresh fruit toppings in place of syrups. Read those labels. Most of us are being overdosed on high fructose corn syrup.

STEP 15: FISH, SOY PRODUCTS, NUTS, WHOLE GRAINS, LEGUMES, AND EGG WHITES ARE LEAN, HEALTHY PROTEIN SOURCES.

STEP 16: START YOUR DAY WITH A GLASS OF WATER. DRINK AT LEAST SIX TO NINE GLASSES A DAY. MORE IF YOU'RE PHYSICALLY ACTIVE.

STEP 17: HIGH FIBER FOODS HELP CURB THE APPETITE.

CHAPTER SIX

EATING

Diets that don't satisfy your hunger won't work in the end. You can't rely entirely on "will-power." It's there some days; some days it's not.

What works is eating health-promoting foods you enjoy. With the knowledge you've gained thus far, you can take any mouthwatering recipe and turn it into a healthy one by substituting good fats for bad fats, whole grain products for refined carbohydrates and by making smart protein choices. You'll become slimmer and healthier. Here are a few suggestions for healthy meals.

*****

BREAKFAST

Before every meal drink a glass of water and swallow a fish oil capsule for the omega-3 fatty acid and to slow down the absorption of glucose. Before breakfast, take a tablespoon of insoluble fiber like psyllium seed in glass of water.

The "Everything-Healthful-Omelet," call it Frittata if you want, is made with three egg whites or egg substitutes cooked in a pan coated with olive oil spray. Pour the eggs over simmering chopped or diced vegetables: onions, peppers, cauliflower, broccoli, chickpeas, tomatoes, kidney beans, mushrooms, garlic and artichokes. Yuck, you don't like broccoli? Chopped it up into tiny, tiny pieces and your taste buds won't notice it in the omelet.

If you're strapped for time, you can buy your vegetables already chopped or pick up a package of stir-fry. You can also buy egg substitute products with the vegetables already in the mix. I chop up a three-day supply of omelet vegetables at a time and store them in a baggies in the refrigerator.

Be inventive and add as many nutritious vegetables as you can. For flavor and texture, add chunks of tofu or a chopped-up soy hotdog. You can buy pre-cooked cubes of turkey to add to your omelet. Salmon, shrimp, or crab also goes well in an omelet. Experiment until you come up with your own "Everything-Healthful-Omelet" that satisfies your taste buds. Make sure your protein choices are smart ones.

If you're a "bacon and eggs" person, blot off as much bacon fat as possible with a paper towel. If you must have greasy bacon, spray it with some olive oil or grape seed oil after blotting. Alternatively, use soy bacon or soy sausage. They contain mostly unsaturated fats and only a few grams of carbohydrate.

For toast, use whole grain bread with at least three grams of fiber per slice. Toast lightly. You can lower your cholesterol by using Benecol or Take Control spreads.

Watch out for those lead-heavy muffins and super-sized bagels. French toast with butter and syrup has enough calories and carbs to be explosive. Ideally, all baked goods should be made with whole grain flour and unsaturated oil. It's hard to find healthy foods when you're eating on the run. However, it's your health. If you can't find a bakery that supplies healthy goods, buy from a health food store.

If you are not getting your vegetables in the morning, drink a few ounces of vegetable juice with your breakfast. Some vegetable juices contain sugar or high fructose corn syrup, so limit the juice to three ounces or less. Better yet, take time to make that vegetable-rich omelet.

Have a cup of green, black, or white tea. **Warning:** don't drink it piping hot. Hot drinks can damage the esophagus (swallowing tube) and predispose to cancer. British women drink their tea very hot and they have high rates of esophageal cancer. It's the heat and not the tea that's the problem.

Tea is an excellent choice to go with any meal. Green tea is loaded with antioxidants and lowers the risk for some cancers. It's believed to destroy cancer cells that have already formed. It's also touted for preventing tooth decay and bad breath.

Coffee has been the subject of numerous studies and I'm not aware of any correlation between coffee drinking and heart disease. The more coffee is studied, the better it looks. Of course, too much caffeine from any source can make you jittery, interfere with sleep, irritate the stomach lining and cause palpitations. I've known people who go into rage when they get too much caffeine. Then, there's "coffee breath" and stained teeth.

A study of eight thousand men in Hawaii found that drinking coffee lessens their chances of developing Parkinson's disease, a common degenerative condition of the brain that results in uncontrollable shaking, poor control of muscles and other symptoms. The Harvard Health Professionals Follow-Up Study 2003 newsletter states, "men who consume moderate amounts of caffeine (equivalent to one cup of regular coffee per day or more) have half the risk of Parkinson's disease than men who do not consume caffeine."

The caffeine in tea, chocolate and other products may also be protective of the brain cells involved in Parkinson's disease. Studies indicate that drinking coffee can reduce the risk of Type II Diabetes, colon cancer, gallstones and cirrhosis of the liver. More studies are needed. In the meantime, have a cup of tea or coffee with your meals.

If you are a cereal person in the mornings, use "whole grain" cereals and pick one with lots of fiber. Spike it with blueberries or mixed berries to make it even more wholesome. If you opt for the cereal, leave off the toast and bakery products to avoid overloading on carbs. Choose a cereal without hydrogenated or partially hydrogenated fats. Do not eat pasta and cereal on the same day.

If you choose grapefruit for breakfast and you're taking medications, check with your doctor or pharmacist. Grapefruit interacts with many medications including cholesterol-lowering pills, heart medicines and tranquillizers.

If you want pancakes now and then, that's no problem. Use a whole grain pancake mix or soy flour, skim milk or soymilk and egg whites without the yolks to cut down on total fat and calories. Use fruit extracts for flavoring. Add chopped nuts, blueberries, mashed sweet potatoes, or chips of dark chocolate to the batter. Use fruit or sauce toppings in place of syrup.

*****

LUNCH

Eating should be a pleasurable social event, conducted with style, conversation, grace, and enjoyment. Although, who has the time? My doctor's office is a mom and pop operation. My wife, a schoolteacher turned receptionist-business manager-nurse-counselor, hates to cook. For more than thirty years, our lunches have been heat and eat. Over the years, we learned to make them healthy. It's amazing how quickly one can prepare a healthy meal with only 30 minutes to eat, clean up and get back to work.

We buy whole-dressed wild Alaskan salmon, cut it into filets, bag it and store it in the freezer. You can thaw and cook a salmon filet in 3 to 4 minutes in the microwave, or broil it for 5 minutes in the oven. With a little lemon and marjoram, it tastes ever bit as good as grilled salmon.

While I cook the salmon, my wife makes a lettuce and spinach leaf salad. She slices the tomatoes and I cooked them for 40 seconds in the microwave to rupture the tomato cells and release the health-promoting, cancer-preventing, eye-protecting lycopene. We use Paul Newman's "olive oil and garlic" and "vinegar and red wine" salad dressings. I use these Paul Newman dressings because I like the ingredients. My wife uses them because she's secretly in love with Paul Newman. However, watch out for the ranch dressing, too many calories and fat grams.

Sometimes we have a turkey white meat sandwich on whole wheat bread. We pile on the lettuce and tomato. Mustard is a free condiment—no bad fats, no bad carbs, no high fructose corn syrup and only a few calories. I often fix myself a "prostate burger," a sandwich designed to protect me from that male gland whose only function is to cause trouble.

A "prostate burger" is really a soy burger, microwaved and covered with chopped green onions or scallions, tomatoes, mustard and a little garlic salt. I fold it up in a lettuce wrapping for a breadless sandwich. Tasty, if a little messy, but healthy and slimming. The soy burgers I use have only one-half gram of saturated fat.

When really hurried, we call ahead to the local restaurant. Our salads and main dishes are waiting for us when we rush in with our bottle of Paul Newman. When I can't get away from the office, I eat an apple or orange along with natural peanut butter on whole wheat and wash it down with soymilk.

Your lunch can be anything from a gourmet meal to a bowl of kidney beans with onions. Keep it healthy with smart protein choices and always be on the look out for those omnipresent refined carbs, high fructose corn syrup and bad fats. Make sure you get your vegetables and fruit with every meal. Frozen brussels sprouts can be thawed and cooked in the microwave in minutes.

A quick fruit fix, bursting with antioxidants, can be prepared in seconds. Microwave a bowl of frozen Berry Medley containing blueberries, raspberries, strawberries and blackberries. It takes a mere 40 seconds to make this delicious, healthy treat. Add a little fat-free yogurt if you want.

Eating salads at a fast food restaurant can be tricky. The fat grams in some fast food salads are nearly half the FDA's total recommended daily allotment of 65 grams. To lower the fat content of salad, pick off the croutons and bacon.

Watch out for the salad dressing. Some fast food dressings are real killers, heavy with calories and fat grams. If you're not sure about the dressing, ask about the ingredients or look them up in a food manual. Better yet, take your own vinegar and red wine Paul Newman with you.

Why a vinegar dressing? Acetic acid, the active ingredient in vinegar, slows the absorption of glucose from the digestive tract, blunting insulin spikes. Don't go swigging down straight vinegar. Acetic acid in excess can eat the enamel off your teeth.

*****

DINNER

After a long day at work, most of us look forward to a sumptuous dinner. It's often the most pleasant time of a day when family members gather to enjoy conversation and food. The lyrics of an old Johnny Cash tune, "Suppertime" go something like this, "...some of the fondest memories of childhood are woven around suppertime, when mother used to call from the back steps of the old home place, 'come on son, it's suppertime...'"

So that suppertime doesn't become a dangerous diet time, do some advance planning. Use fish or poultry frequently as a main dish. Try soy chicken Jambalaya, soy hash, or any of number of soy meat substitutes as a protein choice. Avoid the frying pan. Cooking fish and meat at high temperatures can create heterocyclic amines, chemicals associated with some cancers. Oven-roast or bake most dishes. Microwave meat until it's 80% done before barbequing, frying, or broiling to decrease those nasty heterocyclic amines.

If you haven't had your seven to nine servings of fruit and vegetables by suppertime, do an "Everything-Healthful-Salad," the counterpart to the "Everything-Healthful-Omelet." Use green leafy vegetables, tuna or salmon, red grapes or strawberries, kidney beans, mushrooms, apple slices, melon, broccoli, cauliflower and onions in the medley.

For dessert, try a berry medley, a soy smoothie (soy milk with soy powder), tofu ice cream, non-fat yogurt or soy yogurt.

Richard A. Uhlig, D.O.

*****

FOREIGN CUISINE

The French Food Connection has intrigued doctors for years. The French diet is chock-full of cheeses and rich sauces. The French eat flaky croissants, creamy pastries, buttery ladyfingers and they drink alcoholic beverages with their meals. Yet, they are slimmer than we Americans. How can this be?

The French eat less than we do and take longer to do it. Undoubtedly, they're pitchforkers who savor the flavor. They don't snack as much as we do and their food portions are smaller. We Americans demand our money's worth. We've become a culture of super-sized candy bars, giant sandwiches, mega-drinks and king-size meals.

Keep the following serving guidelines in mind: A typical 3-ounce serving of meat should be no bigger than a deck of cards. An average serving of mashed potatoes is ice cream scoop size. A serving of fruit or vegetable, baseball size. A serving of pasta, half a tennis ball—remember, use whole grain pastas.

When eating out, call ahead to see what items are on the menu and to check on the ingredients. Ask the waiter not to bring a breadbasket to the table. Insulin levels soar if you eat bread on an empty stomach. When you order, ask that half your meal to be packed in a doggy bag before it's served. You'll have tonight's dinner and tomorrow's lunch for one price and you halved your calories. Children in China won't starve if you don't clean your plate.

Citizens of Greece, Italy and the 14 other countries that border the Mediterranean Sea live longer and have less heart disease and cancer than most other peoples of the world. The so-called "Mediterranean Diet" is rich in grains, fruits, vegetables, olive oil, beans and nuts. It's moderate in fish and low in meat and diary compared to the American diet. Asians, also known for longevity, eat pretty much the same diet minus the olive oil, but more soy.

Should we all run out and eat Italian? Wait a second. Eating out is like a box of chocolates; you're never sure what you're getting. Americanized Italian and Old World Italian foods are not always the same. Real Italian pizza has less crust and the dough is made with olive oil. Some American eggplant parmigiana servings can be over 1,000 calories, same with spaghetti and meatballs. Watch out for deep fried zucchini sticks and calamari. I do not recommend any deep-fried foods.

Some Italian restaurants stick with the Old World cuisine. Find out. Ask about the oils and other ingredients. If the waiter stares at you like you're from another planet, just tell him you want to get slim and stay healthy. If they toss you out on your neck, pick yourself up, brush yourself off and go try some real ethnic foods.

The Japanese have the longest healthy life expectancy in the world. So try some sushi, chicken yakitori, or some of the soy dishes. Indian food is extremely tasty with lots of vegetables. If you eat Chinese ask for brown rice. One of the healthiest, best tasting meals I have ever eaten was at a Lebanese restaurant.

Foreign cuisines generally use more fish and vegetables and less red meat than we do. Additionally, portion sizes are smaller.

If you're in a bind over what's for dinner? Think seafood, but be cognizant of the warnings about contaminants. Try grilled Portobello caps with shrimp, using olive oil, lemon juice, tomatoes and basil leaves in the recipe. It's low calorie and low carbs. Wild salmon is always a winner. Try shrimp with one of those tasty sauces made with olive oil, vinegar, garlic and cayenne pepper. Here's an idea, shrimp with a fruit relish of mangoes, pineapple and lime peel.

*****

THE CALORIE CRUNCH

We said diets that severely restrict calories work in the beginning, but usually can't be sustained. Then we said that a diet that doesn't satisfy hunger doesn't work. So, what's a person to do? In the 1930's, it was discovered that rats fed low calorie diets lived 30% longer than rats fed a normal diet. Of course, the rats had nothing to say about it. People do.

A low calorie diet lowers cholesterol, reduces the amounts of free radicals and protects against insulin resistance. Starvation does the same thing. However, who wants to starve to live longer! We can accomplish the same thing without torturing ourselves and we can do it by eating the right foods: fruits and vegetables, whole grains and smart protein selections. Instead of counting calories, count on eating the right foods. You'll lose weight, keep it off, stay healthy and live longer.

STEP 18: HAVE SOME CAFFEINE EVERYDAY. ONE OR TWO CUPS OF COFFEE IS FINE. GREEN TEA IS A GREAT HEALTH FOOD.
STEP 19: BEFORE EATING OUT, CALL AND CHECK OUT THE MENU AND INGREDIENTS.
STEP 20: REDUCE SERVING SIZE AND EAT SLOWLY. PITCH-FORK.

Live Thin, Live Long

CHAPTER SEVEN

SNACKING

Most of us snack. It's natural as breathing. I read somewhere that Americans consumed 30 million pounds of snack foods during the last Superbowl. Snacking isn't all bad; it can give you an energy boast and prevent overeating at mealtime. However, munching on chips, pretzels and rice cakes will shoot up insulin levels. Prepare your own snacks to avoid refined carbs and bad fats.

Here are some suggestions:

1. Make a smoothie in the blender with frozen berries and low-fat yogurt.

2. Cut up some vegetable sticks and fruit slices.

3. Have an apple or an orange.

4. A slice of watermelon.

5. One tablespoon of natural peanut butter and wash it down with soymilk.

6. Have some low fat cheese or soy cheese.

7. Make some breadless lettuce-wrapped hors d'oeuvres with low-fat turkey meat or chunks of soy burger.

8. Drink a tofu and low fat yogurt shake.

9. Have a bowl of air-popped popcorn.

10. Mixed nuts.

11. Red grapes.

12. Sardines

A piece of antioxidant-packed, semi-sweet dark chocolate makes a great snack. Dark chocolate lowers the blood pressure and protects the heart by thinning the blood. It's the *dark* chocolate that's loaded with antioxidants, not the milk chocolate. If you're a chocoholic, watch out. Chocolate products contain saturated fats, sugar and gobs of calories. No bingeing.

If you can't eat just one piece of chocolate or one tablespoon of peanut butter, then leave them completely alone, don't keep them in the house. Too much of a good thing can be fattening.

What about dip and chips? For chips use whole grain tortillas microwaved with olive oil. Use flavored hummus or guacamole as a dip.

Make cookies with whole grain flour or soy flour. Add ground almonds to the cookie batter. A small bowl of whole grain cereal can serve as a snack. Granola and protein bars are okay if you're exercising, but read those labels. Drink a glass or two of water before you snack. You'll eat less and feel full quicker.

I had a patient who couldn't lose weight, because every time he walked by the refrigerator he opened it. His kitchen was close to the bedroom, so he had no trouble making nighttime raids on the refrigerator. He ended up putting his refrigerator in the basement, which cut down on his snack trips and gave him daily stair-climbing exercise. He lost 30 pounds.

A heavy "snacker" is like an addicted smoker. When I was a smoker, my wife ruled I couldn't smoke in the house or in the car. One cold, wintry night, she noticed I wasn't in bed. She found me in the garage, standing barefoot on the cold concrete floor next to my Volkswagen, puffing on my pipe.

If you're an addicted snacker, make snacking as difficult as possible. Don't keep your favorite snack foods at home. If you go out and buy them, buy only one snack hit at a time. The more often you have to go out, the less likely you are to over-snack.

Over-snacking has two components: snacking on the wrong foods and snacking too often. Work on limiting your snacks to between meals and a small evening snack. If you cheat, be a healthy cheater, use celery, carrots, natural peanut butter, a few nuts, grapes, or berries.

If you must have that rare ice cream fix, go out and eat it, so there's no ice cream in the freezer, beckoning. Ice cream should not be an everyday treat. I recommend a cup frozen low fat yogurt, which has $1/25^{th}$ the calories of a banana split.

STEP 21: LIMIT YOURSELF TO TWO OR THREE SNACKS DAILY. AVOID SUGARY TREATS AND JUNK FOODS. MAKE YOUR OWN HEALTHY SNACKS.

Live Thin, Live Long

CHAPTER EIGHT

APPETITE

Hunger is a complicated neuro-hormonal drive that demands satisfaction. It's your body calling out for nourishment. Survivors of World War II concentration camps reported that when on starvation rations, hunger pains never go away. They spent their days and nights behind barbed wire dreaming and fantasizing about food. Although diets that sharply restrict calories work in the beginning, hunger eventually defeats them. That's why smart food choices that satisfy your hunger will allow you to lose weight and keep it off for the long term.

As we pointed out, willpower is fickle; you can't depend on it. It's better to use those simple diet substitutions (whole grains in place of refined carbs, good fats in place of bad fats, smart protein choices), which will allow you to eat enough to satisfy your appetite, while keeping you thin and healthy.

Excessive hunger and weight gain can be caused by undiagnosed diabetes, thyroid conditions and medications such as tranquillizers, antidepressants, hormones, arthritis pills, and steroids. Serious eating disorders such as bulimia and anorexia nervosa require medical intervention.

For most of us, excessive hunger and food cravings are not caused by any underlying physical condition. Just the same, we shouldn't blame ourselves for a lack of will power. Overeating and over-snacking often have an emotional basis. We eat when bored, when uneasy in social situations, when angry and when lonely. Eating becomes a way of coping. Many of us tend to fill the emptiness in our lives with food. Emotional food carvings can often be controlled by waiting them out or by satisfying them with an activity other than eating: calling a friend, writing a letter, taking a walk, or cleaning out a closet.

*****

Mary Duncan was 40 years old and weighed 290 pounds. She was a binge eater who had tried diet pills, yo-yoed at Weight Watchers and took antidepressants for low self-esteem and depression. She came to me because her periods were irregular and heavy and she complained of having no energy. She was found to be anemic. A pelvic sonogram showed multiple uterine tumors. I referred her to a gynecologist who refused to remove her diseased uterus until she lost 80 lbs.

I asked Mary to keep a food diary and record her feelings when food cravings hit. She often ate when she wasn't hungry and often at night when she couldn't sleep. Her diary revealed her eating triggers were emotional. She ate when she felt lonely or sad. Her foods of choice were sugary snacks.

I had her substitute whole grains for refined carbs and sugars. I asked her to prepare healthy snacks in advance of food cravings and to get the ice cream, cookies, chips, candies and other comfort foods out of the house. Once she was off the refined carbs, sugars and bad fats for two weeks, her food cravings lessened. Next, I recommended exercise, but her painful knees made it difficult. She finally settled on a recumbent, stationary bicycle. After six weeks, she stopped her antidepressant.

Mary lost the 80 pounds and her surgery was successful. She continued to lose weight and went from muumuus to size 14 dresses. She has kept the weight off, because, like a reformed alcoholic, she takes life one day at a time. She knows she is not cured, but her food cravings are under control. She goofs occasionally, but jumps right back into the program. She's slowly easing into a healthy lifestyle.

*****

Triggers in the environment can set off a snack-attack: a football game on TV, a movie, a game of cards, a telephone conversation, unsettling news and even sitting down with a good book. On the job, we often snack with fellow workers and eat whatever the group eats. The trick is to bring your own healthy snacks to the job and don't rely on others for snacks. Some of us eat when bored or under tension. Others use food as a substitute for affection and companionship.

If you identify those situations and triggers that set off your cravings, you're more likely to control them. Drinking water, exercising and just taking a walk can often ward off a craving. I had one patient who knitted to keep her hands and mind busy whenever she felt the urge to snack. It worked for her and she filled her husband's closet with fine sweaters.

Excessive insulin levels from eating refined carbohydrates causes a rebound low blood sugar, which in turn causes a ravenous hunger. That's why shortly after a sugary snack, or after eating a bag of chips or pretzels, we're suddenly hungry again. By replacing those foods with whole grain products, fruits, vegetables, healthy "UN" fats and smart protein choices, you can avoid "rebound hunger," satisfy your appetite and control your cravings.

STEP 22: IDENTIFY THE TRIGGERS AND SITUATIONS THAT CAUSE YOU TO OVEREAT. KEEP A FOOD DIARY AND WRITE DOWN YOUR FEELINGS AND REASONS FOR SNACKING.
STEP 23: REMOVE COMFORT FOODS FROM THE HOUSE. REPLACE THEM WITH HEALTHY SNACKS.

Richard A. Uhlig, D.O.

CHAPTER NINE

DON'T MEASURE, DON'T SMOKE

Weigh no oftener than once a week. Watching your weight fluctuate a few pounds from day to day can be discouraging. Your clothes often tell you how you're doing.

I knew a overweight patient who kept meticulous charts on the dimensions of her anatomy: waist, neck, arms above the elbows, buttocks, breasts, thighs and legs. She bought a house-load of exercise equipment, tried diet drinks, diet pills, wore a step-meter and even went out of town to buy food especially prepared for her. She jumped from one fad diet to the next and never settled into a sustained healthy lifestyle.

She yo-yoed on her weight and in the end, she gained. Her weight gain didn't bother her as much as her measurements. She was upset over her girth size and burgeoning arms. Repeatedly, I talked to her about meaningful lifestyle changes and smart food choices, but she was only interested in diet pills and quick fixes.

Many people pre-occupied with their body image become hooked on the measuring tape. They believe their bodies are imperfect in some way. That's why plastic surgeons are so busy. This is not to say that plastic surgery's out of the question for everyone. Quite the contrary. If you can improve your appearance, your self-image and your confidence by having your jowls lifted or the bags under your eyes reduced — do it. However, if you don't make the necessary lifestyle changes that will keep you slim and fit, you're wasting your time and money.

Our genes determine our basic body shape and little can be

done about that. Some people work for years at tightening their abs and butts. If they would only eat smart and did simple walking exercises, their bodies would take on a naturally healthy shape. My mother had a saying that said a lot, "Pretty is as pretty does."

*****

Jack was a 60 year-old warehouse clerk who smoked a pack of cigarettes every day. He was 5'9" and 240 pounds and he hated being overweight. Jack had quit smoking several years ago and gained 20 pounds. He started smoking again to lose weight. More than anything, Jack wanted to be thin, despite having a naturally stocky, powerful build. He was willing to suffer the consequences of smoking to keep from gaining weight.

His mood vacillated with the readings of the scale. Nothing made him happier than to weigh in a pound lighter than the day before. Any weight gain was an instant downer. His weight, however, kept creeping up and I worried he would have a heart attack.

I convinced him to have some tests. His cholesterol profile was excellent, chest x-ray normal and his treadmill stress test showed no signs of heart disease.

The next time I saw him, he complained of a cough. Chest x-ray this time showed a tiny "spot" in the left lung. The CAT scan was suspicious of a tumor. I referred him to a lung specialist who did a bronchoscope that showed lung cancer. A surgeon did a biopsy, which showed the cancer had already spread. Jack was sent to a cancer specialist who started chemotherapy and radiation treatments.

Unfortunately, the treatments didn't work for Jack. He was dying. In a bizarre sort of way, he was happy he was finally losing weight. He'd step off the scale with a broad smile. "Hey, Doc, I lost another five pounds." Jack never connected the dots. He died weighing less than 150 pounds.

*****

Getting sidetrack with weights and measurements can be a mistake. Forget about the measuring tape and concentrate on a smart, healthy lifestyle. With a little perseverance, you can defeat any bad habit. If you're a smoker and overweight, first stop smoking. Once that habit is under control, then go to work on the weight.

STEP 24: WEIGH NO OFTENER THAN ONCE A WEEK.
STEP 25: IF YOU SMOKE, QUIT!

Live Thin, Live Long

CHAPTER 10

THE DANGER ZONES

This chapter contains bad news and good news. Brace yourself for the bad news. As we grow older, we are more likely to fall victim to diseases. High blood pressure, arthritis, Alzheimer's disease, breast cancer, prostate cancer, lung cancer, blindness, heart attacks and strokes happen most often to people over 50. The older we become, the more we are at risk for these diseases.

HERE'S THE GOOD NEWS—if you're already eating those whole grains instead of refined carbs, getting in your 7 to 9 servings of fruits and vegetables each day, substituting good UN fats for the bad saturated and trans fats and making smart protein choices—you've already reduced your risk for the above mentioned diseases considerably.

The revolutionary findings of "Harvard Health Professionals Follow-Up Study" (HHPF) and other studies have identified many food booby traps associated with disease. Making intelligent, health-promoting food choices can help fend off these threats to our health.

*****

PROSTATE CANCER

An old professor of mine once said, "If a man lives long enough, he'll get prostate cancer." This adage is backed by scientific data. A series of autopsies on men in their eighties who died of various causes showed greater than 70% of them had cancer of the prostate. There are two types of prostate cancer, the aggressive and the non-aggressive. Both can kill you; the aggressive type just does it faster. Some men with non-aggressive prostate cancer never know it and live to a considerable old age.

The Harvard Health Professionals Follow-Up Study (HHPF) 2003 Newsletter reported, "...that high intakes of tomato products were associated with a reduced risk of prostate cancer." The study also found that high intakes of red meat, processed meats and dairy products were associated with a moderately increased risk of metastatic prostate cancer. Metastatic means that the cancer has spread to other parts of the body.

On the other hand, men who regularly consumed three servings a week of salmon, tuna, or sardines had a 40% reduction in the risk of metastatic prostate cancer. The HHPF 2003 newsletter stated, "Although we need to do more work to determine the specific factors, our results strongly support recommendations for men to reduce intake of red and processed meats and instead to rely more on fish, poultry and plant sources as their main sources of protein."

The 1995 HHPF newsletter reported, "...animal fat was directly related to risk of advance prostate cancer."

The HHPF reported in 1999, "Consumption of more than two glasses of milk per day versus none was associated with almost twice the risk of advanced and metastatic prostate cancer." The increased risk of prostate cancer due to dairy products may be related to the calcium contained in those products. Supplemental sources of calcium were also associated with higher risk.

For men over 50 years old calcium supplements may increase the risk of prostate cancer. On the other hand, for both men and women, calcium may reduce the risk of colon cancer. Calcium supplements in women and some men are of value in treating and preventing softening of the bones.

If a man's brother or father has had prostate cancer, that man is at increased risk for getting it. If you are black, the risk is increased. Studies have indicated that increased levels of insulin-like growth factors are associated with the development of prostate cancer. If you're an "apple shape" with insulin resistance, your risk may be increased. Yet, another reason to avoid refined carbs.

A study of the drug Finasteride, trade name Proscar, used to treat benign enlarged prostates and baldness, showed taking Proscar may reduce the risk of getting prostate cancer. In general, if you exercise and stay active, your risk for almost any cancer is decreased.

Selenium, a chemical element used in semiconductors and by our body's enzyme systems, when taken as a supplement, has been shown to reduce the risk of prostate and other cancers. Usual dose is 200 micrograms a day; a higher dose may lead to toxicity. Fish oil may also reduce the risk of prostate cancer.

Prostate cancer is a threat to every man. Positive steps can be taken to reduce that risk. Every man 40 or over should see his doctor for a yearly digital rectal exam and a blood test for prostate cancer called the PSA.

*****

BREAST CANCER

Most breast cancers occur after menopause. Risk factors include family history of breast cancer, not having children or having them late in life, not breast feeding, early onset of menstruation, late onset of menopause and cysts or benign tumors of the breast.

In postmenopausal women, weight gain and diabetes are associated with an increased risk for breast cancer — yet, another reason to avoid refined carbs.

The *Brigham and Women's Hospital Nurses' Health Study* showed that women beyond menopause who consumed one and a half alcoholic drinks a day increased their risk for developing breast cancer. If they took hormones for over 5 years and drank, the risk doubled. For some unknown reason, white women living in affluent suburban areas are at increase risk. For women who drank, a daily multivitamin with folic acid may offer some protection.

The *Nurse's Health Study* reported in the *Journal of the National Cancer Institute* that women who eat a diet high in animal fats increased their risk for breast cancer. Dietary risk factors for prostate cancer in men and breast cancer in women are similar.

Both men and women over 50 should reduce their intakes of animal fats by consuming less red meat and dairy products. They should increase fruits, vegetables and whole grains in the diet; and eat more fish, soy, and nuts.

Women over 50 should avoid alcohol or reduce consumption to one drink or less in any single day and no more than four drinks a week. Taking fish oil capsules daily may offer some protection against breast cancer by favorably changing the ratio of omega-3 to omega-6 fatty acids. It's risky for anyone over 50 to be overweight or to smoke.

*****

COLON CANCER

Colon cancer is the second leading cause of cancer deaths after lung cancer. Ninety percent of the cases occur in people over 50. Most colon cancers began as polyps, small growths that protrude into the lumen of the colon and that's why colonoscopy works well for early detection. Any rectal bleeding should be brought to the attention of your doctor.

Several studies have shown that insulin resistance increases the risk of colon cancer. Increased insulin levels activate an enzyme called COX-2, which promotes the development of polyps, which can give rise to cancer. The good news is that aspirin and some arthritis medications block the COX-2 enzyme. Taking aspirin every day over a long period reduces your risk for colon cancer. Taking folic acid can also reduce the risk. Both aspirin and folic acid also protect the heart. Markedly reducing or eliminating refined carbs in the diet is essential for controlling insulin resistance.

Reduced intakes of calcium increase the risk of colon cancer. Taking calcium supplement makes good sense for women. However, for men, as we pointed out earlier, calcium may increase the risk of prostate cancer. Men should discuss the risks and benefits of taking calcium with their doctors. The HHPF 2003 newsletter states that for men, "…current evidence suggests moderate intakes of calcium (approximately in the range of 800-1000 mg/day) may be most prudent."

More than two alcoholic drinks a day doubles your risk for colon cancer, but this risk can be lessened by taking high doses of folic acid.

The HHPF study uncovered a connection between smoking in earlier life and developing colon cancer in later life. The study also showed that consumption of red meat and fat increased one's risk of getting colon cancer.

To reduce your risk for colon cancer, do the following: Replace refined carbs with whole grain carbs. Reduce your intake of trans fats and red meat. Eat more vegetables and fruit. Avoid tobacco. Reduce alcohol intake to one drink or less a day (no more than 4 drinks a week). Take a folic acid supplement. Take aspirin daily, but consult your doctor if you have a history of bleeding or stomach problems. Take calcium supplements—for sure for women, men need to weigh the risk.

*****

LUNG CANCER

Lung cancer is the number one cause of cancer deaths in America. If you are a smoker, or have been a smoker, you are at increased risk. Smoking causes about 80% of lung cancers. Other causes include radon, asbestos and exhaust fumes. The average age of a lung cancer victim is around 60. Survival rates are low because only one case in five is caught early. If you are a smoker, quit NOW!

Quitting tobacco will definitely reduce your risk for lung cancer, colon cancer, heart disease, stroke and blindness due to macular degeneration. Also, avoid secondhand smoke, diesel exhaust and other noxious fumes. Check your house for radon.

Flavanoids, plant substances found in citrus fruits and teas may offer some protection from lung cancer. Selenium, which we said was protective for prostate and breast cancer, may offer some protection from lung cancer. Apple skins contain high levels of a compound called Quercetin, a potent anti-oxidant believed to possibly reduce the risk of lung cancer.

In summary, DON'T SMOKE. If you do smoke, QUIT NOW. Avoid fumes and second hand smoke. Eat foods containing flavanoids—oranges, tangerines and teas. Eat apples, take selenium and exercise.

*****

HEART ATTACK

This is the number one killer in America and other industrialized nations. Heart attacks strike over million people in the United States very year and nearly half are fatal.

A heart attack happens when one of the small arteries that supply blood to heart muscle suddenly clogs and the involved portion of the heart muscle dies. If you have chest discomfort or other symptoms of a heart attack, call 911. The longer you wait, the greater is your risk of sudden death or crippling heart damage.

The risk factors for heart attack include family history, smoking, high cholesterol and high blood pressure. For years, men were at higher risk for heart attacks than women. Today, it is the number one killer of women.

If you smoke, stop. Have your blood pressure checked, if it's elevated, get it treated. Start exercising, but it's a good idea to get a treadmill stress test first. Have your blood lipids (cholesterol and triglycerides) checked and if elevated, treated. Avoid saturated and trans fats. Take fish oil. Eat lots of fruits and vegetables and use smart protein choices (fish, soy, nuts, whole grains, and legumes).

*****

MACULAR DEGENERATION

Macular degeneration is the leading cause of blindness after 50. It affects the part of the retina crucial to central vision. Even if it doesn't blind you, it can interfere with driving, reading, watching TV and recognizing people. Contributing factors are heredity, smoking, high blood pressure and a diet high in saturated fats, cholesterol and salt.

Eating fish (salmon, tuna, mackerel) at least twice a week helps prevent macular degeneration, as does eating seven to nine portions of fruits or vegetables each day (especially green leafy and brightly colored vegetables). Stop smoking, exercise regularly and wear sunglasses outdoors. New drugs are being tested that might aid in preventing and treating macular degeneration.

*****

CATARACTS

Cataracts, a clouding of the normally transparent lens within the eye, are common after 50. Cataract victims often feel as if there's a film over their eye. Vision is reduced and blindness can occur. Prevention may not be possible, but the development of cataracts can be slowed. Wear a brimmed hat and sunglasses to block sunlight. Stay away from tanning booths. Eat vegetables and fruits high in vitamin C. Take vitamin E supplement. If you have Diabetes or high blood pressure, keep them under good control. If you smoke, QUIT!

*****

ARTHRITIS

Osteoarthritis, a deterioration of joint cartilage, affects over 20 million Americans. It can progress to complete destruction of a joint. The cause is not clear and neither is prevention.

Obesity contributes significantly to arthritis of the knees. An extra 10 pounds of weight produces an extra 50 pounds of force on knee joints with each step. Repetitive strain and injury to a joint can cause arthritis.

Much has been written about diet and arthritis and all the exorbitant claims and diet cures proven false. However, a healthy diet with lots of vegetables and fruits makes sense. Eating fish or taking fish oil capsules reduces inflammation in some forms of arthritis.

When your joints hurt and swell, exercise is not very appealing. Yet, regular exercise can improve joint pain. If your joints are inflamed and swollen, you can reduce the stress on them by exercising in water.

STEP 26: LIMIT ALCOHOLIC BEVERAGES TO FOUR DRINKS A WEEK OR LESS; NEVER MORE THAN TWO DRINKS IN ANY ONE DAY FOR MEN, AND ONLY ONE DRINK IN ANY ONE DAY FOR WOMEN. MAKE RED WINE YOUR DRINK OF CHOICE.
(A DRINK EQUALS 12 OUNCES OF BEER OR 5 OUNCES OF WINE OR 1 1/2 OUNCES OF HARD LIQUOR)
STEP 27: USE FISH, SOY, NUTS, WHOLE GRAINS, BEANS AND LEGUMES AS MAJOR PROTEIN SOURCES.

CHAPTER 11

AGING

Growing older and aging are not the same thing. Growing older is normal; aging is pathological. One of the purposes of this book is to help you grow older without aging. Growing older means living a vigorous and energetic life, staying engaged, benefiting from experience and anticipating and embracing new experiences.

Aging is an abnormal decline in bodily functions occurring with time. When one ages, the skin loses tautness, wrinkles and spots happen. Muscles lose strength. Joints stiffen. Memory slips. Vision dims. Hearing fades. Remember the handsome, dashing, high school fullback who at the twentieth class reunion looked like Wilford Brimley on a bad mustache day.

To understand what causes aging, we need a couple of definitions.

Free Radicals are highly destructive chemicals produced as a by-product during the normal chemical activities of our cells. Free radicals attack and damage our cells in the same way air oxidizes iron to rust or turns a peeled apple brown. If left unchallenged, these chemicals break down our tissues, damage our arteries, induce inflammation and attack our DNA. In short, free radicals cause aging and disease. Smoking, exposure to radioactivity and eating the wrong foods promote the production of free radicals.

Antioxidants are substances that destroy free radicals. They are the rust inhibitors of the body. Most come from the vegetables and fruits we eat. Selenium, quercetin, lutein, lycopene and vitamins A, C and E are antioxidants. By mopping up free radicals, antioxidants prevent tissue damage and halt the abnormal changes that lead to aging. Other plant substances such as phytochemicals work with antioxidants to keep our tissues healthy and to protect us from disease.

In the war between "free radicals" and "antioxidants," aging occurs when the free radicals are winning. We can change the tide of battle by cutting out refined carbs and bad fats and replacing them with whole grains, nuts, fruits, vegetables and fish (salmon, tuna, and sardines).

As we grow older, our bodies produce more free radicals and make fewer natural antioxidants to combat them. Therefore, it's important to take supplements of vitamins C and E, fish oil and selenium daily.

Here are some proven ways to stay young and vigorous, despite the years.

*****

EXERCISE

The benefits of regular exercise are well known. Exercise increases mobility, strength and endurance. Circulation improves with exercise. We are more mentally alert when we exercise regularly. Exercise reduces blood pressure, decreases bone loss, cuts the risk for many cancers and protects us from heart disease and strokes. Recent studies show that if you have cancer, you're more likely to survive if you exercise.

The problem with exercise like so many other things is *sticking with it*. The old axiom, "No pain, no gain," is not true. Only three hours of exercise per week can strengthen the heart and reduce the risk of cancer. It doesn't have to be strenuous. Something as simple as brisk walking or riding a stationary bicycle yields great benefits. A little exercise is better than none at all.

If you find an exercise you enjoy, so much the better. Start slow. Don't make excuses for not doing it. Get into a routine.

When a vacation or some unexpected event disrupts your exercising routine, get right back to it at the first opportunity. You'll look and feel younger for the effort.

Lifting weights and I'm not talking about Olympic-size barbells, but something you can lift easily, will increase your muscle mass. Since muscles burn calories at a greater rate than fat, you'll lose excess pounds faster. Consult a personal trainer or someone knowledgeable before starting a weight lifting program. Be careful and always warm-up. Injuries can bring any exercise program to a standstill.

When watching TV, do it from a moving treadmill or a stationary bicycle. At commercials, instead of sticking your head in the refrigerator, do some simple calisthenics.

In our busy lives, it is often difficult to find the time for exercise. Here are some ideas. When you take the trash out, walk all the way around the house—two or three times. Park your car at the far end of the parking lot. When shopping, walk briskly and use the mall as a track. Skip the bus and walk downtown. Use a push lawnmower. Shovel your own snow (beware of severe exertion in extreme cold). Hand-deliver those inter-office memos. Take the stairs instead of the elevator. Do isometrics at your desk. Play catch with the kids. Do standing push-ups against the kitchen counter. Take breaks from the computer to stretch, do crunches, or to take a short walk.

*****

SKIN CARE

Ultraviolet light from the sun and the tanning booth causes wrinkles, age spots and skin cancers. Fluctuations in body weight along with gravity cause sagging. Cigarette smoking causes wrinkling and other effects. Alcohol consumption, except for red wine, is associated with an increase in skin cancers. Rosacea, a thickening and reddening of the facial skin, has also been linked to alcohol.

Age spots can be lightened with "fade" creams from the doctor. Fine wrinkles can be treated with topical medications or laser. A physician should check out any pigmented skin spots you may have for possible melanoma, a deadly form of skin cancer.

Wear sunscreens with SPF of 15 or above when exposed to sunlight between 10 a.m. and 3 p.m. and wear a brimmed hat, sunglasses and long sleeves. Drink plenty of water and use moisturizing creams or lotions to prevent drying of the skin, especially in the winter.

The foods you eat affect the health of your skin. Lycopene, found in tomatoes and watermelon, protects the skin from sun damage. Salmon, fish oil, green tea, prunes, green leafy vegetables and flavanoids found in citrus fruits also protect the skin from sun damage and prevent skin aging.

One should keep in mind that a little sun exposure is good. We get most of our vitamin D from sunlight. Vitamin D has been shown to be protective against many types of cancer. Others sources of vitamin D are fish (especially salmon, herring, and cod liver oil) and vitamin supplements.

*****

STOP SMOKING!

Smoking promotes aging inside and out. On the inside, smoking narrows arteries, which reduces blood flow to organs and increases free radicals in the tissues. It inactivates enzyme systems essential to normal cell function. It elevates blood pressure and damages the lungs, blood vessels, heart and eyes. Smoking is the leading cause of lung cancer.

On the outside, smoking results in wrinkles, furrows, and an unnatural graying of the skin. The skin loses suppleness and sags. There's only one thing to do—QUIT!

If you smoke first thing in the morning and right after meals, you're probably physically addicted. If you need help to quit, join a support group. Nicotine gum, nasal spray and patches are available. Your doctor may prescribe a medicine that reduces tobacco craving and softens the rigors of withdrawal.

Squeezing a rubber ball whenever you get the urge to smoke can help. Aromatic capsules with eucalyptus can act as a substitute for the tobacco taste, so can chewing gum. For some people puffing on fake cigarettes help. Do whatever it takes, because smoking not only ages you, it can kill you. If you backslide, don't get discouraged. Most ex-smokers had quit several times before they succeeded.

Don't worry about weight gain when quitting tobacco. First, conquered the nicotine demon.

*****

MIND AND MEMORY

Intellectual abilities and aptitudes do not normally decline with the years. Information processing may slow and memory banks may become so full that it takes longer to recall a name. Impaired thinking after 50 is usually due to untreated high blood pressure, poorly controlled diabetes, or Alzheimer's disease.

The risk factors for high blood pressure and Type 2 Diabetes include obesity, smoking, eating refined carbohydrates and consuming saturated and trans fats. If you reduce these risks, you can keep your mind working efficiently, no matter your age.

It's a myth that memory deteriorates with the years. Forgetting is no more common at 70 than at 37. There's just more memories and stored information to handle at 70. Some people remember past experiences better than recent ones. This may be because past experience had a more profound effect on them. You remember vividly the pageantry and excitement of your first football game. However, you can hardly remember which teams played last Saturday on TV.

*****

ALZHEIMER'S DISEASE

Alzheimer's Disease, a form of dementia, is not a normal part of growing older, although the risk of getting it increases with age. The early symptoms of Alzheimer's are loss of recent memory, misplacing common objects, getting lost and becoming irritable for no apparent reason. Severe personality changes can occur and proceed to apathy and death.

Damage due to free-radicals undoubtedly play a role in Alzheimer's, hence the rationale for using Vitamin E to help prevent the disease and to slow its progression. As mentioned earlier, one study showed eating fish regularly reduced the risk of getting Alzheimer's. Aspirin and some arthritis medications may also cut the risk by reducing inflammation.

A recent study indicated that brain damage caused by strokes play an important role in some cases of dementia. This goes along with observations that repeated head injuries have been associated with the development of Alzheimer's. Cholesterol-lowering medications called "statins" may prevent small, undetectable strokes and thus help prevent Alzheimer's. People who were physically and mentally active in their middle years are less likely to develop Alzheimer's later on.

You can reduce the risk of getting Alzheimer's by controlling blood pressure, reducing cholesterol, severely limiting the amount of saturated and trans fats in our diets, eating more fish and replacing refined carbohydrates with whole grain foods. Eating healthy works every time.

*****

MENOPAUSE

A sharp decrease in a woman's sex hormones occurs at menopause. Eating soy products rich in phytoestrogens may alleviate the night sweats and hot flashes. Lubricants like K-Y and Replens help with vaginal dryness. Calcium supplements aid in preventing softening of the bones. Being overweight after menopause put women at high risk for stroke, heart attack and cancer. Smart nutrition is an absolute "must" at menopause.

*****

STAY ACTIVE

Stay active mentally, physically and sexually.

Negative cultural attitudes concerning sex and older people are commonplace. It's bunk. When men grow older, they often have more control over orgasm, prolonging the sexual act. Postmenopausal women have a greater sense of sexual freedom since they no longer worry about pregnancy. Erectile dysfunctional is a treatable condition. Simply losing excess pounds can improve sexual function. If you're losing interest in sex, hormones may be the problem. Consult your physician.

To stay active mentally, stay active socially. Consider joining an exercise group, reading club, dance club, or a service club. Get involved in church activities and community projects. They can fill the void left by retirement. Take a class, find a job, or volunteer your services and experiences to your old firm or a new company. You'll feel better staying engaged. Stay informed and keep an open mind to new ideas. Read. Take up a cause.

If you can't think of a cause to champion, try this one. Wild salmon is one of the healthiest foods in world, but it could disappear or become too polluted to eat. Fourteen hydroelectric dams on the Columbia and Snake Rivers have blocked natural salmon runs in the Northwest. Federal and State governments and the hydroelectric industry have given lip service to the problem, but little has been done.

Worse, mercury pollution from coal-burning power plants, factories and incinerators end up in our waters and accumulate in fish and in the people who eat fish. Our government has recently eased controls on power plant polluters and others instead of tightening them. Write your congressperson, join an activist group, put an editorial in the local paper, get connected on the net, SPEAK OUT!

STAY YOUNG

When your hair or beard turns gray making you look older than you think you are, dye it. If it turns out badly and your hair glows under florescent lights like the aurora borealis, try a different product next time. Many people are timid about such things. Not too many years ago, people thought it pretentious to wear sunglasses. Live as young as you feel. Be daring. If painted acrylic fingernails boost your self-image, do it. If your eyelids are droopy water bags, get 'em fixed.

Stay engaged and stay active. Go for it!

STEP 28: TAKE A MULTIVITAMIN WITH FOLIC ACID DAILY.
STEP 29: TAKE SELENIUM 200 MCG. DAILY.
STEP 30: TAKE VITAMIN C 500MG. DAILY AND VITAMIN E 400 UNITS DAILY.
STEP 31: EXERCISE A MINIMUM OF 3 HOURS A WEEK.
STEP 32: WHEN OUTSIDE DURING PEAK SUN HOURS, USE SUNSCREEN, WEAR A BRIMMED HAT AND SUNGLASSES.
STEP 33: STAY ACTIVE.

Chapter 12

Think, Plan, and Succeed

If you've read this far, that's good evidence you're dedicated to losing weight, keeping it off, staying healthy and living longer. You've learned some strategies for handling tough food situations, for avoiding food booby-traps and for making smart food choices. You now actually have the knowledge and the power to prevent disease and to live thin. What's left?

One last obstacle — staying motivated.

Eating healthy is a lifelong commitment and there will be "setbacks." You'll be on your own out there in the food world, bombarded by commercials, surrounded by fast food restaurants that don't give a rap about your health or your girth. These saturated fat hucksters are in it for profit and they're caught up in a taste and super-sizing war. They spend millions on advertising and hawking plastic toys to kids in hopes of sucking in the whole family.

Food manufacturers will saturate you with trans fats and high fructose corn syrup if you let them, and they'll mislead you with labeling tricks. Even the government's food pyramid, our guide to healthy eating, is so flawed, that it's dangerous. I recently talked with a physician consultant for the new food pyramid. His message, don't expect any major improvements. The special interests and food lobbyists are again clamoring to get their products on the lower rungs of the USDA's new triangle.

Family, friends and co-workers can influence your food choices. There'll always be those special events to be celebrated with tempting, high-caloric, unhealthy treats. Periods of loneli-ness and boredom can have you reaching for the refrigerator door. We all have moments of weakness and we all experience those turns and twists that can totally disrupt our day.

You will have setbacks.

However, that's all right. Setbacks are part of developing the "Live Thin, Live Long," lifestyle. Look at them as an opportunity to re-motivate, to come up with new strategies for handling tough food situations. You can conquer failure by thinking about your mistakes and by thinking ahead.

Learn to solve potential problems beforehand. Where will you be eating tomorrow? What will you eat? Who will you be eating with? Make a mental list of those restaurants where you can eat healthy food.

Don't go to the grocery store on an empty stomach. Keep a working grocery list in the kitchen, on the fridge door. Don't trust your memory. Be sure to read those labels when you shop. Read-ing labels is our only protection from those dangerous food sub-stances such as trans fats.

Write down your food mistakes. Be painfully honest about them. I've known people who swear they've been perfect with their food choices. When I see them at the smorgasbord of the local restaurant filling their plates, it's apparent they suffer from "food amnesia."

Many people honestly don't remember what they've eaten during the day. Eating has become automatic as breathing for them. They get so lost in a dinner conversation, in a TV show, or in the newspaper, they don't even realize they're stuffing their face.

Practice being conscious of your food each time you pick up your fork. Think about it when you chew and swallow.

If you have trouble remembering what you've eaten during the day, write it down in a food journal. Go over your daily food fare like a bookkeeper totaling up the ledger at the end of the day. If you know where you've been, you'll have better control over where you're going.

Sometime during the day, in the shower or tub, when you're

all alone, think back on the day's setbacks and successes. Be kind to yourself, knowing you'll do better tomorrow. Visualize your solutions. This thinking, this being conscious about your food life will lead to a healthy lifestyle. It all begins with thinking about it.

Sometimes the scales or your clothes will tell you that you're doing something wrong. You've been too busy to think, to plan and now you're up five pounds. This happened to a patient of mine. An accountant overloaded with work and racing toward a tax deadline, he stopped planning his meals and began sending out for fast food, which he ate at his desk. After a long day at work, he felt too exhausted to exercise in the evenings.

I asked him to keep a food journal and to begin planning his meals again. He started doing isometrics at his desk and walking to the post office each day as well as to work. In three weeks he had the lost those five pounds and met his work deadlines with no problems.

We've demonstrated some food strategies in this book. The best strategies will be those you come up with yourself. By constantly thinking about your food life, you'll discover solutions for your particular eating problems. Reading and re-reading this book and the summaries at the end of the chapters will help keep you on track.

With constant vigilance, you will achieve your goals. You will lose weight, keep it off, stay healthy and live longer.

1. REPLACE REFINED CARBOHYDRATES WITH WHOLE GRAIN PRODUCTS. AVOID SUGARY SNACKS AND SUGARY SOFT DRINKS.
2. IF YOU HAVE CEREAL FOR BREAKFAST, LEAVE OFF THE TOAST.
3. DON'T EAT CEREAL AND PASTA ON THE SAME DAY.
4. DON'T EAT A SANDWICH AND PASTRY ON THE SAME DAY.
5. EAT 7 TO 9 OR MORE SERVINGS OF FRUIT AND VEGETABLES A DAY.
6. TAKE A FISH OIL CAPSULE BEFORE MEALS.

7. EAT BEFORE GOING TO SOCIAL DINNERS AND EAT A HEALTHY SNACK WHEN YOU GET HOME.

8. BE A PITCHFORK EATER.

9. GIVE YOURSELF TWENTY MINUTES FOR A FOOD URGE TO PASS.

10. USE ONLY LEAN CUTS OF RED MEAT, NO MORE THAN 3 TO 6 OUNCES IN ANY ONE DAY. TRIM AWAY ALL FAT. AVOID PROCESSED MEATS. YOU DON'T HAVE TO EAT MEAT EVERY DAY.

11. USE SOY MILK OR SKIM MILK IN PLACE OF WHOLE MILK AND 2% MILK.

12. BUY LOW-FAT OR FAT-FREE CHEESE OR SOY CHEESE.

13. ROAST OR BAKE INSTEAD OF FRYING. NEVER DEEP-FRY.

14. READ THOSE LABELS. AVOID TRANS FATS. REDUCE SATURATED FATS TO A MINIMUM.

15. FISH, SOY PRODUCTS, NUTS, WHOLE GRAINS, LE-GUMES AND EGG WHITES ARE LEAN, HEALTHY PROTEIN CHOICES.

16. START YOUR DAY WITH A GLASS OF WATER. DRINK AT LEAST SIX TO NINE GLASSES A DAY. MORE IF YOU'RE PHYSICALLY ACTIVE.

17. HIGH FIBER FOODS HELP CURB THE APPETITE.

18. HAVE SOME CAFFEINE EVERYDAY. ONE OR TWO CUPS OF COFFEE IS FINE. GREEN TEA IS A GREAT HEALTH FOOD.

19. BEFORE EATING OUT, CALL AND CHECK OUT THE MENU AND INGREDIENTS.

20. REDUCE SERVING SIZE AND EAT SLOWLY. PITCH-FORK.

21. LIMIT YOURSELF TO TWO OR THREE SNACKS DAILY. AVOID SUGARY TREATS AND JUNK FOODS. MAKE YOUR OWN HEALTHY SNACKS.

22. IDENTIFY THE TRIGGERS AND SITUATIONS THAT CAUSE YOU TO OVEREAT. KEEP A FOOD DIARY AND WRITE DOWN YOUR FEELINGS AND REASONS FOR

SNACKING.

23. REMOVE COMFORT FOODS FROM THE HOUSE. RE-PLACE THEM WITH HEALTHY SNACKS.

24. WEIGH NO OFTENER THAN ONCE A WEEK.

25. IF YOU SMOKE, QUIT!

26. LIMIT ALCOHOLIC BEVERAGES TO FOUR DRINKS A WEEK OR LESS; NEVER MORE THAN TWO DRINKS IN ANY ONE DAY FOR MEN AND ONLY ONE DRINK IN ANY ONE DAY FOR WOMEN. MAKE RED WINE YOUR DRINK OF CHOICE. (A DRINK EQUALS 12 OUNCES OF BEER OR 5 OUNCES OF WINE OR 1 ½ OUNCES OF HARD LIQUOR)

27. CAN'T SAY THIS ONE ENOUGH. USE FISH, SOY, NUTS, WHOLE GRAINS, BEANS AND LEGUMES AS MAJOR PRO-TEIN SOURCES.

28. TAKE A MULTIVITAMIN WITH FOLIC ACID DAILY.

29. TAKE SELENIUM 200 MCG. DAILY

30. TAKE VITAMIN C 500 MG. DAILY AND VITAMIN E 400 UNITS DAILY.

31. EXERCISE A MINIMUM OF 3 HOURS A WEEK.

32. WHEN OUTSIDE DURING PEAK SUN HOURS, USE SUN-SCREEN, WEAR A BRIMMED HAT AND SUNGLASSES.

33. STAY ACTIVE.

34. THINK, PLAN AND SUCCEED.

35. LIVE THIN, LIVE LONG.

Live Thin, Live Long

Printed in the United States
43599LVS00001B/58-60